THE ETHICS OF HEALTH CARE RATIONING

THE ETHICS OF HEALTH CARE RATIONING

John Butler

CASSELL

Cassell

Wellington House
125 Strand
London WC2R 0BB

370 Lexington Avenue
New York
NY 10017 – 6550

First published 1999

British Library Cataloguing-in-Publication Data
A catalogue record for this book is available from the British Library.

ISBN 0–304–70581–0 (hb)
    0–304–70582–9 (pb)

Typeset by York House Typographic Ltd
Printed and bound in Great Britain by TJ International Ltd, Padstow, Cornwall

Contents

Preface

Although this book is entirely my own work and I am solely responsible for the errors and imperfections that it surely contains, I have been greatly helped and encouraged by a number of friends and colleagues without whose continuing interest the book may not have been brought to completion. I would like to express my particular gratitude to Sandro Limentani, whose understanding of moral philosophy and whose practical experiences in public health have left their mark in very many places in the text. I am deeply appreciative of his generosity in reading and commenting upon the entire text and in sharing so many of his ideas in areas where I had so few of my own. Robin Gill has given me a great deal of intellectual, practical and moral help, and to him too I am grateful. I would like also to thank Peter Taylor-Gooby, Sally Gordon-Boyd, Gillian Paterson, Cally Vaile, Seth Edwards and Ruth McCurry. The shrewd comments of members of the Archbishop of Canterbury's Advisory Group on Medical Ethics were also of great value to me at a critical stage in my thinking.

Those who, apart from Sandro and Robin, gave me the greatest help cannot be named. They are the front-line NHS staff who kindly agreed to talk to me about their own perspectives on ethics and rationing and who gave me permission to reproduce their 'stories' in Chapter 6. Certain details of their stories have been changed or rendered anonymous in order to protect their identities, but they are nonetheless of considerable value in grounding the debates about rationing in the realities of life at the cutting edge of medical and nursing care. Indeed, I think that the stories are perhaps the most valuable part of the book. It is relatively easy to theorize about health care rationing from the comfort of a university office. It is much more difficult to cope with it as an ever-present feature of one's daily work. In gathering the stories that are told in Chapter 6, I was deeply impressed with the integrity and commitment of these people, struggling as they all were with the daily need to squeeze a quart of care from a pint pot of resources while always striving for the highest professional standards in their work. If these stories are anything to go by, the NHS is very well served by its staff at the front line of care, and I think that their views and experiences should be heeded every bit as much as those of outside commentators such as myself. I am sorry that I cannot name the story-tellers – but that was the deal!

JOHN BUTLER
UNIVERSITY OF KENT AT CANTERBURY
DECEMBER 1998

Introduction

The inconsistent triad

Fashions come and go, in public sector services as much as in any other area of human endeavour, and health care is no exception. If effectiveness and efficiency were the fashionable ideas of the National Health Service (NHS) in the 1970s and 1980s, scarcity and rationing were the buzzwords of the 1990s and may continue to be the smart talking-point into the new millennium. A hatful of texts on rationing in the NHS appeared in the 1990s, most of them drawing upon the wisdom of a common group of expositors and covering broadly similar territory (Bowling, 1993; Frankel and West, 1993; Smith, 1993; Tunbridge, 1993; Harrison and Hunter, 1994; Malek, 1994; House of Commons Health Committee, 1995; Maxwell, 1995a; Mullen, 1995; Royal College of Physicians, 1995; Stewart *et al.*, 1995; Coast, Donovan and Frankel, 1996; Klein, Day and Redmayne, 1996; Lenaghan, 1996; New and Le Grand, 1996; Honigsbaum, Holmström and Calltorp, 1997; New, 1997; Hunter, 1997). Nor was the debate about scarcity and rationing located only, or even mainly, in the UK or in the context of the NHS. Similar dialogues, engaging similar ideas and expressions, were known to be under way at much the same time in America (Strosberg *et al.*, 1992), Sweden (McKee and Figueras, 1996), Holland (Dunning, 1992), New Zealand (Hadorn and Holmes, 1997), Norway (Hansson, Norheim and Ruyter, 1994), Denmark (Danish Council of Ethics, 1996) and Israel (Chinitz *et al.*, 1998). Indeed, in many respects the arguments were more explicit and focused elsewhere than within the UK, perhaps reflecting the continuing unwillingness of UK governments publicly to acknowledge the existence of the problem.

The language may vary from one country to another and from one discipline to the next, but the issue is essentially the same: how best to square the proverbial welfare circle (George and Miller, 1994). How can resources be matched to needs, or needs to resources, in politically acceptable ways? Weale (1998) presents the dilemma as an inconsistent triad, a set of three propositions of which any two are compatible but which together form a contradiction. A classical illustration of the inconsistent triad is the sign on the garage forecourt:

> We provide three kinds of service – cheap, quick and reliable. You can have any two, but you can't have all three. If it's cheap and quick it won't be reliable. If it's cheap and reliable it won't be quick. And if it's quick and reliable it won't be cheap.

In the case of health care, Weale proposes that the three material components of the triad are 'comprehensive care', 'high quality care' and 'care available on the basis of people's need rather than their ability to pay'. We can have any two together but not all three; and it is possible to see in broad terms where different countries have made the trade-off. Health care systems that are organized on market lines (of which the private sector in the US is the exemplar) offer comprehensive and high-quality care, but only to those who can afford it. By contrast, publicly funded health care in the US, most famously through the Medicaid programme in the State of Oregon, offers high-quality care on the basis of need, but the package is limited. And examples of the third kind of trade-off are found in systems that reflect the command and control economies of the former Soviet bloc, which offer comprehensive care on the basis of people's need, but the quality is patchy.

The high political profile enjoyed by the NHS has discouraged successive British governments from acknowledging the reality of the inconsistent triad. Publicly, at least, the image has been upheld of an NHS that remains faithful to the vision of its creators, providing comprehensive care of a uniformly high quality to all those in need of it. 'The NHS', promised Prime Minister Blair in the foreword to his government's White Paper on the NHS in 1997, 'will get better every year so that it . . . delivers dependable, high quality care based on need, not on ability to pay . . . [It will] produce better care. Care when you need it. Care of uniformly high standards' (Department of Health, 1997a). Although the noise of political rhetoric has failed to still the debate about scarcity and rationing, it has confined it somewhat to the professional margins of public life. Managers, doctors, nurses and above all academics have enjoyed a sustained and extensive perambulation through the area, conferring and writing about health care rationing in all its facets for a decade or more. Yet precisely because the political stage has for long been largely off-limits, the impression may have grown that rationing is a technical matter to be discussed and resolved in secret places only by those who know about marginal utility, the prudential life-span account and quality-adjusted life years, not by patients, citizens or electors.

Such a view, if it is held, is mistaken. It is mistaken for at least two reasons. Firstly, there are no technical solutions to the inconsistent triad in health care – though technology can certainly help in elucidating the range of options. There is no uniquely 'correct' way of matching resources to needs, or needs to resources. If there were, it would by now have been disclosed. To search for the 'right' solution is to bay for the moon, for the problem cannot be resolved in any universally acceptable way. It can only be debated with the greatest possible clarity and openness to ensure that decisions, when they have to be taken, are reflective of informed moral opinions. Secondly, the problem is inherently contestable because it touches upon social, political and economic values about which people not only care but also disagree. To limit the debate about health care rationing only to the *cognoscenti* is to restrict the range of values it can encompass. To be sure, it may demand a degree of technical expertise from those who wish to engage in it, but the dialogue needs to be structured and conducted in a way that lays it open to a wide spectrum of informed opinion. To suppose that we can escape the dilemmas of rationing by retreating into a simple world where values are redundant and technical fixes abound is, as Weale (1998) insists, to cast a veil of deceit over the choices that must be made.

This book is about scarcity and rationing in health care. It proceeds from the assumption that rationing is concerned with values as well as techniques, and that the debate about rationing in the NHS ought therefore to proceed across as wide and diverse a canvas as possible. Rationing is a moral issue as well as a managerial and clinical one. The first chapter sets the scene by reviewing the principal landmarks in the British debate. It describes the gap between needs and resources, the principles that could be followed in bridging it, and the methods by which it has been done in the UK and, to some extent, elsewhere. The chapter concludes that, while rationing *per se* is not unethical, the ways in which it is done may raise questions of an ethical nature.

The next four chapters explore the ways in which the moral bases of health care rationing have been handled in the literature. They all address the common question of what we understand by a fair distribution of health care resources in situations where they are inadequate to meet the needs of all, but they do so from differing perspectives. Chapter

2 focuses on the personal qualities of those who are competing for resources, Chapter 3 on the structural ordering of services, Chapter 4 on the processes involved in the rationing of resources and Chapter 5 on the outcomes of rationing. Chapter 6 presents a series of 'stories' told by some of those who are engaged, in one way or another, at the sharp end of rationing in the NHS. They describe the extent to which and the ways in which rationing affects their daily work with patients, and they reflect upon some of the ethical issues thrown up by their experiences. The final chapter draws a number of themes together by reflecting on the moral principles and practices of health care rationing in the NHS.

1

Scarcity and rationing

The gap between supply and demand in health care: theory

The history of medicine discloses the infinite capacity of doctors to do ever more – and ever more expensive – things for their patients (Porter, 1997). Medicine is both a limitless art and a costly science. Enoch Powell's observation about the generous capacity of people to absorb the ministrations of their doctors was an early expression of this insight, carrying the particular authority of a then Minister of Health. 'Every advance in medical science', he wrote, 'creates new needs that did not exist until the means of meeting them came into existence, or at least into the realms of the possible' (Powell, 1966, p. 26). The point was well illustrated in the final illness in 1975 of the Spanish Fascist leader, General Franco, when his doctors used every weapon in their armoury to keep him alive.

A defibulator [sic] attached to his chest shocks his heart back to normal when it slows or fades. A pump-like device helps push his blood through his body when it weakens. A respirator helps him breathe, and a kidney machine cleans his blood. At various times in his 25-day crisis General Franco has had tubes down his windpipe to provide air, down his nose to provide nourishment, in his abdomen to drain accumulative fluids, in his digestive tract to relieve gastric pressure, and in his left thigh to relieve the pressure of blood clots . . . He has undergone emergency surgery twice – once to patch a ruptured artery to save him from bleeding to death, the second time to remove most of an ulcerated and bleeding stomach for the same reason. He has taken some 15 litres of blood transfusions. (United Press Agency, quoted in Porter, 1997, p. 700)

Such aggressive treatment in the face of poor survival odds may not be all that unusual: similar scenes are likely to be enacted in every major hospital on every day of the week. Whether it is ethically justifiable, not least when it is done at the expense of younger patients requiring major elective surgery, is a question that must be deferred for the time being. Yet the case of General Franco is a graphic reminder of the gulf that exists between the capacity of patients to receive medical care and their ability to pay for it. For whether care is organized as a tax-funded service that is free at the point of use or as a commercial enterprise for which people pay either directly or through insurance, it is simply not possible to offer the full spectrum of clinical possibilities to every patient at every stage of life. The cost would be unsustainable, whether it fell on citizens as tax-payers or on patients as fee-payers.

It is this simple observation about the contradiction between clinical possibility and economic affordability that underlies the idea of an inescapable gap between supply and demand in health care. Resources are always and intrinsically scarce in relation to the things that people want. As Fuchs puts it, 'it is hardly news that we cannot all have everything that we would like to have, but it is worth emphasising that this basic human condition is not to be attributed to "the system" or to some conspiracy, but to the parsimony of nature in providing mankind with the resources needed to satisfy human wants' (Fuchs, 1974, p. 4). It is, in part, a matter of the natural limits that all societies must place on the amount they can afford to spend on health care in relation to everything else. However much health care may be valued, it cannot be valued so far above all the other services of public life (education, defence, housing, communications, investment, income maintenance, and so on) that nothing will ever be spent on such alternatives until each and every health care need has been fully met. The Royal Commission on the NHS had no difficulty accepting the view put to it by one of its witnesses that 'we can easily spend the whole of the gross national product on the NHS' (Royal Commission, 1979, para. 21.5); yet successive UK governments, charged with spending the nation's resources in a prudent manner, have never seen fit to allocate more than about 7 per cent of the gross national product to caring for the health needs of the people.

More than this, as Powell (1966) understood, the nature of health care is such that supply often generates its own demand; and to spend more on the provision of care is often to do no more than to stoke the fires of further demand. We have only to think of psychotherapy, hormone replacement therapy, transplantation and graft surgery, antibiotic drugs, screening techniques, joint replacements – the list is endless. Since to conquer one peak is merely to reveal yet others to climb, we cannot assume that a doubling or even a trebling of the volume of resources allocated to the NHS would close the gap between supply and demand. It was, in part, the failure to realize the dynamic nature of the relationship between supply and demand that led the founding fathers of the NHS into seriously false errors about the self-limiting nature of health care expenditure.

The gap between supply and demand in health care: evidence

The theory is sustained by evidence. A pioneering study by an American economist and physician in 1983 attempted to measure the extent to which people's needs for hospital care in the UK were failing to be met (or, in their terminology, the extent to which treatments were being rationed) because of inadequate resources (Aaron and Schwartz, 1984). The study was based on the assumption that people's needs for each of eleven specific treatments were being fully met in the US, and that any lesser level of provision in the UK would be indicative of their being rationed. Of the eleven treatments, three were found to be provided at essentially the same rate in both countries and were therefore judged not to be subject to rationing in the UK: treatment for haemophilia, radiotherapy and bone marrow transplantation. The remaining eight treatments were 'clearly rationed in Britain when compared with per capita levels of consumption in the United States' (*op. cit.*, p. 28). These were: X-ray examinations, the treatment of chronic renal failure, total parenteral nutrition, CT (computed tomography) scanning, intensive care, coronary artery surgery, hip replacement and (though to a lesser extent) chemotherapy for cancer. Aaron and Schwartz concluded that, in comparison with the US, these treatments were being rationed in the UK largely because of a shortage of resources. Doctors carry out fewer of these treatments in the UK because they have more limited resources.

Aaron and Schwartz's analysis has been criticized as naïve and even arrogant (Miller and Miller, 1986). The uncritical assumption that the provision of hospital care in the US is 'right', and that any deviation from it is prima facie evidence of rationing in the UK, has little justification. On the one hand it ignores the extent of explicit rationing that exists in the US through the denial of needed treatment to the millions of

American citizens who are uninsured or inadequately insured (Dixon, 1992). On the other it ignores the extent to which clinical custom and practice in the US are driven to extremes by the expectations of patients, by the fear that doctors have of being sued for inadequate care, and by the influence over their clinical judgement of the fees they can earn from unnecessary care (Glaser, 1970). There is an important distinction between what *can* be done for patients and what *should* be done for them even in as wealthy a country as the US (Kassirer, 1998); and a former President of the Royal College of Physicians has criticized Aaron and Schwartz's work for failing to understand that British doctors may actually be more discerning than their American counterparts and more critical of the potential benefits of certain treatments (Hoffenberg, 1987).

Nevertheless, Aaron and Schwartz's study, conducted at a time when the notion of health care rationing was rarely on the agenda of public or professional debate, exposed the likely extent to which patients in the UK were being denied the treatments that, in a more prosperous context, they might have received. Whether desirable or not, more could – and probably would – have been done for them if the resources to do so had been available. This was true, Aaron and Schwartz surmised, not only in the treatments they selected for particular examination but in other areas of care also. Based upon their observations of the NHS, they identified the kinds of services and treatments that were, in their view, most likely to be rationed by a shortage of resources. These included services that depended upon specialized capital equipment and staff, the care of older people, treatments that are costly in relation to the medical benefits they yield, and those which may succeed in prolonging life only at the expense of a sharp reduction in its quality (*op. cit.*, pp. 110–11).

An avalanche of evidence since Aaron and Schwartz's study in 1983 has merely reinforced their message. There is a substantial and sustained shortfall in the provision of renal replacement therapy for new patients in the UK (Mallick, 1993). Some cancer patients are receiving much less intensive therapy than others with apparently similar conditions (Priestman *et al.*, 1989). Patients above a certain age have been denied intensive care (Zimmerman, quoted in Charnley, Lewis and Farrow, 1989). Alcoholics have been turned away from liver transplantation programmes (Moss and Siegler, 1991). Effective chemotherapy for ovarian cancer is being rationed by health authorities (Royal College of Physicians, 1998). Rates of coronary bypass surgery are lower in Britain than in many other developed countries, even among angina patients whose symptoms would be relieved by the treatment (Smith, 1991b). Fewer than three per cent of couples who might benefit from assisted conception are receiving treatment (Winston, quoted in Smith, 1991b). Health authorities are quietly dropping certain services from the menu of those they can afford to provide through the NHS (Klein, Day and Redmayne, 1996). Expensive drugs are not always available to those who may benefit from them (Rous *et al.*, 1996). Dedicated units for the rehabilitation of elderly patients following a stroke are patchily distributed throughout the country (Young, Robinson and Dickinson, 1998). The list is huge and many more examples can be found in the 'stories' told in Chapter 6. The gap between supply and demand is there. It is real, not imagined.

The avoidability of the gap

Nevertheless, the question persists of whether the gap may be avoidable (Heginbotham, 1997). Both economic theory and practical experience suggest that it is not. The health care needs of an increasingly elderly and demanding population, coupled with the ingenuity of medical science in finding ever more complex and costly ways of meeting them, are always likely to exceed the economic capacity of any country to satisfy them. This was certainly the view taken by the Conservative government in 1995 which, in evidence to the House of Commons Health Committee, was clear that 'there will always be a gap between all we wish to do and all that we can' (Department of Health, 1995). Although a contrary stance was adopted by the Labour government in 1997, promising as it did an NHS that would deliver high quality care to all the people wherever and whenever it was needed (Department of Health, 1997a), the conventional wisdom is otherwise. The examples are many.

'Almost all of those who spend any time studying this subject', stated the *British Medical Journal* in an editorial in 1996, 'recognise that people have always been denied potentially beneficial treatments and they always will be, no matter how much is spent on health services' (Smith, 1996b, p. 1553). The editorial was triggered by the manifesto of the Rationing Agenda Group (RAG), a consortium of academics, clinicians and health service managers united in their views about the inevitability of rationing and committed to making it work in ethical and democratic ways (New, 1996). In the following year a similar view was expressed by an influential Working Party made up of representatives of the Medical Royal Colleges, the British Medical Association, the National Association of Health Authorities and Trusts and the National Health Service Executive.

> [We] agree with . . . other observers that the gap between resources and demands in the NHS will persist . . . It seems unlikely, in view of

the demographic and technical pressures and public expectations, that the gap will narrow significantly. It is therefore inevitable that there will be difficult choices in the provision of health care for the foreseeable future. (Academy of Medical Royal Colleges *et al.*, 1997, para. 3.4)

Later that year the President of the Royal College of Physicians rammed the message home yet again to the wider readership of *The Times* (Alberti and Lessof, 1997). 'There is no longer any country in the world, however rich, which can afford to provide all its citizens with access to the increasing range of services, medical procedures and drugs which are becoming available.'

Goliath has not, however, been allowed to roam unopposed. The David in this particular encounter is the Anti-Rationing Group (ARG), another (but appropriately smaller) consortium of academics, clinicians and health service managers. The ARG was formed in the wake of the much-publicized case of Jaymee Bowen (known, before her name was allowed to be divulged, as Child B), a young girl with advanced cancer whose health authority in 1995 refused to pay for innovatory treatment that might have extended her life (Watt and Entwistle, 1996). In the course of the judicial review of her case, Mr Justice Laws said in the High Court that health authorities 'must do more than toll the bell of tight resources . . . they must explain the priorities that have led them to decline to fund [a particular] treatment'.

Heartened by these words, the ARG began to examine the gap between supply and demand not from the conventional assumption that the cost of health care is bound to increase, but from the alternative premiss that health care expenditure should always be rational (Roberts, 1995). By 'rational' the Group meant that no costs should be incurred unless a number of criteria were met: the service in question must have been defined and specified, its clinical effectiveness must have been agreed, its optimal method of delivery must have been established, the required volume of the service must have been measured, and its cost must have been calculated. At first, the Group claimed that, of the total budget of the NHS, about 40 per cent was spent on services that currently met these criteria of rationality; 30 per cent on services that could soon do so; and 30 per cent on services that patently failed to meet them. Later the Group was able to test its calculation through an examination of the purchasing plans of eight health authorities in England and Wales (Roberts, 1996). They found that just over a fifth of all hospital and community care services bought by the authorities were failing to meet the criteria. Among the wasteful practices were the purchase of services that had been inadequately tested for their effectiveness; the over-purchasing of services relative to the demand for them; and the payment of higher prices than were necessary. If such practices could be eradicated, the Group argued, the resources thus released would eliminate the need for rationing in the foreseeable future. The problem, in their view, is not that the NHS is under-funded but that its resources are poorly managed.

An American commentator has pressed the case yet more insistently (Light, 1997). It is, Light contends, downright immoral to assume the existence of an unbridgeable gap between supply and demand in health care, for to do so is to legitimize the rationing of care to patients before all feasible steps have been taken to eliminate waste and inefficiency. Rather, he argues, there is a prior responsibility to examine the ethics of the wider political system that denies a sufficiency of resources in the first place. Waste of the kind identified by the ARG, Light insists, does not merely exist, it reflects a powerful web of interests that prioritize the hidden values of those who manage the resources of the NHS above the needs of the patients. Vested interests of this kind must be subdued before any talk occurs about the need to ration care. 'Our goal', Light concludes, 'should be to minimise the need to ration by eliminating ways that entrenched institutional, political and professional interests lock in waste, not to figure out how to ration fairly in the context of a . . . system with wasted resources' (*op. cit.*, p. 112).

The arguments of Light and the ARG about the avoidability of rationing in the NHS have, in turn, been fiercely rebutted, not least by the public health doctor at the heart of the controversy over the treatment of Jaymee Bowen. Zimmern (1995) derides two of the core assumptions of the Group: that the effectiveness of different services can unambiguously be measured and that the resources released by the elimination of ineffective services (even if they could be identified) would be sufficient to remove the need for rationing. Nor, Zimmern claims, should simple economic ideas of cost-effectiveness be allowed to override other considerations about the range and scale of health services that the country should have. So be it. Yet the arguments of the ARG deserve to be taken seriously. Even if the Group has overstated the savings to be had from a more responsible stewardship of resources, there is power in the idea that the failure to reduce waste and maximize output is both ethically and managerially unacceptable. No rational householder would knowingly persist in buying ineffective goods at inflated prices and then complain that essential services were beyond his or her means. Why should it be any different with a large public corporation?

Sharing out the goods

Market distributions

Whenever the valued things of life are in short supply, ways must be found of resolving one of the most enduring and emotive dilemmas of the human condition: who will get what they want and who will have to go without? In the context of health care, who will get full access to the treatment they require when they are ill and who will receive less than optimal treatment – or even none at all? Aside from contexts of anarchy, where people grab and hold what they want by sheer brute force, the share-out of valued goods and services takes place within rules or customs that are socially negotiated and sanctioned. In broad terms, these arrangements can be thought of as belonging to one of two types: market distributions and rationed distributions.

The market is an ancient and efficient way of regulating the distribution of all kinds of goods and services. It is characteristic of capitalist societies, in which the legitimacy of private ownership holds sway, but the market has also become an increasingly common distributional mechanism for services that are provided by public sector authorities and agencies (Farnham and Horton, 1993). Markets are simple in principle but variable and complex in their operation and control. At the heart of a freely working market is price. If those who produce the goods and services are able to sell their wares at a price, then those who may want them, but who either cannot or will not pay the current price, will fail to get a share of them. Price functions to keep supply and demand in some kind of balance, and in a flexible market prices are continually changing in response to shifts in both supply and demand. Ideally, the price of each item will be set at the level which simultaneously allows the producers to dispose of their stock and the purchasers to acquire the amount they desire.

The persistence and ubiquity of markets attest to their effectiveness and acceptability. They promote efficiency and flexibility, they offer choice and variety to consumers, they encourage risk and innovation, and they generate profits. There is probably nothing that has not been distributed through a market mechanism at some time or in some place. Even many personal services which, in the UK, have been distributed through non-market mechanisms for much of the post-war period, are coming increasingly within its ambit. Pensions, health and social care, income maintenance at times of critical illness, tertiary education, long-term residential and nursing care and the protection of mortgage repayments are all examples of human and financial services that were once the substantial preserve of the public welfare sector but are being distributed increasingly through private markets. Even within what remains of the welfare state, including the NHS, markets of a kind are being used increasingly to regulate the distribution of services (Taylor-Gooby and Lawson, 1993).

Rationing by entitlement

Overshadowing though the market mechanism might be, its dominance has never been total. Some commodities have been, and still are, distributed among those who wish to have them within a socially negotiated framework that takes little or no account of price. It is for this kind of allocatory mechanism that the notion of rationing is best reserved. When goods and services are sold in a market, their allocation is determined largely by their price: they will go to those who are willing to pay the current rate. When they are rationed, it is something other – or substantially other – than people's willingness to pay the current rate that determines the share of the cake they will enjoy.

A broad distinction can be made between rationing mechanisms that depend on rules of entitlement (explicit rationing) and those that depend on the discretion of gatekeepers (implicit rationing). The distinction is by no means hard and fast, and hybrid forms can readily be found. The *Oxford English Dictionary*'s overview of the historically evolving use of the word 'ration' suggests that it may originally have been used in the former sense, denoting a share or portion of a pre-determined size to which each qualified recipient was entitled. From the early eighteenth century the daily ration was the fixed measure of corn given to officers and men in the army and navy. In time, the term was applied to a wider variety of foods than oats and cereals: army rations were described in 1917 as 'standard helpings of various kinds of tasteless food issued by the government to Tommy, to kid him that he is living in luxury while the Germans are starving'. The principle held good, however: the portion was a fixed and unvarying entitlement.

With time, the principle of explicit rationing that began with the military was extended to the civilian population at times of shortage. Mass rationing by entitlement reached its high point in Britain during World War II and beyond, when food and other essential goods that were in short supply were rationed, with fixed weekly allowances for different categories of people. Ration books were issued containing coupons that had to be surrendered to the retailer whenever the designated goods were bought; and when the coupons ran out, the entitlement ceased until the next ration book began. Of course, shoppers still had to pay the price of the goods they wanted, and in that sense the market remained intact. But it was a highly controlled market in which the coupon rather than hard cash determined the quantity of goods that people were able to acquire. Wealthier people could not, officially, use their greater purchasing power to help themselves to a larger share, and even the then Princess Elizabeth bought the dress in which she was married in 1947 with the clothing coupons she is said to have saved.

Unsurprisingly, the notion of 'rations' came to be used as a generic term for things that were shabby or second-rate. In military slang, medals that were awarded automatically, merely for being present at a campaign rather than for distinguished conduct in it, were said to have 'come up with the rations'. Thus Joe Lampton, the archetypal angry young man of the 1950s, 'had no decorations apart from those which all servicemen who served his length of time are given, as they say, with the rations' (Braine, 1957). Unsurprisingly, too, a great deal of time, effort and ingenuity has always been spent during periods of widespread rationing on ways of avoiding the constrictions of the ration book and coupon. Economic transactions conducted 'off the ration' (or, colloquially, on the black market) are part of the folklore of civilian experiences of war. 'We are three spivs of Trafalgar Square, flogging nylons tuppence a pair, all fully fashioned and all off the ration, sold in Trafalgar Square' (Opie and Opie, 1959, page 105).

Rationing by discretion

In contrast to methods of rationing which give a fixed quantum of goods to all those who are qualified to receive them, other methods rely mainly on the discretion or judgment of those who guard the system. Such methods are clearly a type of rationing, for it is something other – or substantially other – than people's willingness to pay a price in the market that largely determines the slice of the cake that each receives. But discretionary methods of rationing give no assurance about the amount that each will receive. At best, people have a general entitlement. An obvious example is the NHS: citizens of the UK have a general entitlement to use the Service, but they have very few explicit assurances about the quantity or quality of care they will receive when they are in need of it. In this and similar cases, decisions about the final allocation of care rest with those in the system who control the flow of patients through it – the so-called 'gatekeepers'.

It is in this more general sense that the notion of rationing is now commonly understood. Rationing, in modern usage, has less to do with the distribution of fixed quanta than with managing the allocatory system in a discretionary way. There is a long history and a voluminous literature about such rationing, particularly in the human and personal services (Ham and Hill, 1984). For present purposes, some general observations will suffice to set the scene for the moral questions to which discretionary rationing processes naturally give rise.

First, the burden of deciding how scarce resources are to be shared among those who want to have them falls largely on the shoulders of the coal-face workers who deal directly with the customers or users of a service. In commercial contexts it is, for example, the garage owner who decides the quantity of petrol that customers can buy at times of national shortage; and in the immediate aftermath of the severe storms that ravaged the south of England in October 1987, it was the local builders who decided the order of priority in which they would fix people's roofs and secure their homes. In the public services the burden falls to social workers, police officers, doctors, nurses, teachers and others whose jobs require them to cope as well as they can with the resources they command. Lacking the certainty of a fixed ration, they must make a continuous stream of bespoke rationing decisions for each new client, patient or pupil they confront.

Lipsky (1980), in his classic American study, termed such people 'street-level bureaucrats'. They work, he argued, with inadequate resources in circumstances where demand will always increase to meet the availability of services, and where they will therefore, by definition, exercise a wide-ranging discretion over the way resources are used. Since they often have neither the time nor the information to make calculated and equitable decisions for everyone with whom they have to deal, street-level bureaucrats develop routines to make their jobs more manageable. One way in which they do this, Lipsky found, is by building up a limited number of stereotypes of their clientele, each with its own distinctive but standard way of management. New clients are then assigned to one of the stereotypes on the basis of a limited number of clues about them, and from this flows a standard mode of meeting their needs.

Secondly, the coping mechanisms developed by street-level bureaucrats raise obvious questions about the bases upon which the stereotypes are founded. Lipsky's evidence led him to some encouraging conclusions. He found the street-level bureaucrats whom he studied to be genuinely motivated by a desire to improve their clients' lives. They were usually highly skilled and experienced professionals, driven as much by the ethical and professional standards of their calling as by the contractual requirements of their employment. Nevertheless, it is of the nature of discretion that personal and other kinds of bias creep into their work, leading to inconsistent, unfair and distorted decisions about the distribution of the resources they control. Some clients evoke excessive sympathy or hostility; some arouse stereotypical responses about the economic value of giving them large amounts of time or attention; some give rise to moralistic judgments about their social worth. Lipsky concluded that bias, however modest, was the rule rather than the exception. The interesting question is not why it occurs but why it sometimes does not.

Thirdly, it is usually of the nature of discretion that it is exercised outside the public gaze. Discretion is, to a greater or lesser degree, cloaked in secrecy. This is particularly true in cases of professional discretion, where confidentiality is an integral part of the relationship between practitioner and client. Sound and sensible though the ethic of confidentiality might be, it conceals the way the rationing process has worked in particular cases. The *outcome* of the process is often knowable in aggregate terms, for example in statistics about the rates of outpatient attendances or hospital admissions among defined groups of the population; but public information is lacking about the *reasons* why individual patients or clients have been treated as they have. Rationing by entitlement, as in wartime, is open and transparent; everyone knows the share of the cake that everyone else has obtained. Rationing by discretion, on the other hand, permits no such common knowledge unless those who exercise the discretion explain what they are doing and why.

Rationing in health care: coping with the gap

The variety of rationing options

In publicly funded health care systems, including the NHS in the UK, little reliance is placed upon market mechanisms as the chosen way of allocating care whenever the needed resources are in short supply. By and large, people's access to publicly funded hospitals, doctors and nurses is not determined by their ability and willingness to pay for the care they need. It follows, then, that if the gap between supply and demand is not to be bridged by price, it must be bridged by some type or combination of rationing.

Various strategies are open to politicians, planners, managers and clinicians in bridging the gap between supply and demand in publicly financed health care systems such as the NHS (Øvretreit, 1997; Hunter, 1997). A distinction is commonly drawn between those that affect the allocation of *resources* or *services*, which are taken at a fairly high level in the system, and those that affect the allocation of *care*, which operate at a lower level. The language may vary, but the idea is similar. Calabresi and Bobbitt (1978), in their analysis of what they call 'tragic choices', draw a distinction between first-order and second-order allocations. First-order allocations determine the total amount of a resource or service that is to be provided; second-order allocations determine the distribution of the total among those who want a share of it. It is a feature of market distributions that the two orders are brought together within a single institutional framework. Thus, to use Calabresi and Bobbitt's example, the market in ships and sealing wax will dictate not only how many (or how much) of these items are available, but also who will acquire them. In rationed systems, by contrast, the first-order and second-order allocations are characteristically taken by separate agencies. The rationing of health care in the NHS, for example, first requires the health authorities or their agents to determine the way the money will be spent between competing services or programmes or client groups, and it then requires those who provide the care to decide how much of it will be used in the care of individual patients. In Klein, Day and Redmayne's (1996) terminology, first-order allocations are concerned with the setting of priorities (macro-rationing) and second-order allocations are concerned with the rationing of care (micro-rationing).

The inherent difficulty of many of the choices that have to be made in health care is intensified, in Calabresi and Bobbitt's analysis, by the inconsistency of values that may occur between macro- and micro-rationing. An obvious example, to which we shall return in Chapter 5, is the conflict that may exist between utilitarian and individualistic approaches to rationing. Utilitarianism broadly seeks to secure the greatest good of the greatest number of people; its outlook encompasses the totality of resources and of people, and it tries to arrive at an allocation that maximizes the well-being of the community as a whole. By its very nature, utilitarianism is likely to appeal most to those who control the levers of macro-rationing – the planners and the managers whose job it is to get the most from the resources they command. By contrast, those who work the levers of micro-rationing – the doctors, nurses and other clinicians – have been trained and socialized in a different school. For them, professional responsibility lies less with maximizing the long-term welfare of the group than with meeting the immediate need of the individual. The doctor's instinct is to save the life of the patient under his or her immediate care whatever may be the opportunity cost of doing so (Hoffenberg, 1987). There is no easy or simple way of reconciling such conflicts of value: they merely compound the tragedy of the choices that may have to be made.

Articulating explicit priorities for health care

A first strategy for managing the gap between supply and demand in publicly financed health care systems is the conscious articulation of explicit priorities for care. It is a strategy that is open both to central government and to local health authorities. If resources do not allow the doing of everything that would be done in an ideal world, then national politicians and local planners can grasp the initiative by prioritizing either the menu of services available or the rules for gaining access to them. By imposing such priorities on those responsible for managing and delivering health care locally, the total cost of services can be brought into a planned and conscious alignment with the annual sums of money that are available. Some services and some client groups will do better than others, but any such inequalities will be deliberate and planned, not arbitrary or accidental.

Service planning of this kind has a long tradition in the NHS, in intent if not always in realization. It was commonplace in the 1960s and 1970s to describe the care of the elderly, the handicapped and the mentally ill as 'priority services' (Department of Health and Social Security, 1976a). In the mid-1970s a new planning system was introduced, complete with guidelines about its intended *modus operandi*, and in 1977 the first fruits of the system appeared. *The Way Forward* set out the ambition of the Department of Health and Social Security to achieve a national pattern of service provision based on national priorities, recognizing that it would require the redistribution of money and manpower between different services (Department of Health and Social Security, 1977). In the event, far too many priorities were listed to provide a national platform for the planned alignment of supply and demand, and most health authorities could do little more than restrain their expenditure on the acute hospitals while investing the small amounts of growth money they received in the designated 'priority services' (Edwards, 1993).

The counterpart document of the early 1990s, *The Health of the Nation*, abandoned the attempt to define priorities in terms of resources, preferring instead to set targets for future levels of morbidity and mortality in a limited number of areas that were major causes of avoidable illness and premature death (Department of Health, 1992). The intention, however, was similar: to provide a more focused approach to the determination of national priorities. Similar also were the hoped-for consequences: patients would get better access to those services thought most likely to move the health of the nation towards the targets set by the government. The successor document of the late 1990s, *Our Healthier Nation*, maintained the principle of setting targets for health, but it was less concerned with the role of health services in meeting them than with the wider social and economic influences on health (Department of Health, 1998). It had more to say about social exclusion and healthier schools and workplaces than about hospitals and health centres.

In the internal market of the early 1990s, central government maintained its influence over the priorities pursued by the health authorities through a series of annual guidelines promulgated by the NHS Management Executive (Klein, Day and Redmayne, 1996, p. 51). The guidelines pressed consistently for progress in pursuing the targets outlined in *The Health of the Nation*, but otherwise they were more concerned with the processes by which health authorities determined their priorities than with the priorities themselves. For example, they emphasized the importance of responding to the needs of patients in an equitable way and of using scientific information to obtain the most effective results from the money that was spent. Yet precisely because the guidelines failed to indicate the volume of resources that health authorities should be aiming to spend on different kinds of services, the political influence of central government over the rationing of services was muted. Instead, the burden of responsibility lay mainly with the executive and non-executive directors of the health authorities and trusts.

The research evidence that has so far emerged suggests that, in spite of the continuing squeeze on their resources and the encouragement they have received from central government to address the issue of priorities in a systematic way, health authorities have largely failed to move their resources from services with lower priorities towards those that are explicitly judged to be of more importance or value (Ham, 1993; Klein, Day and Redmayne, 1996; Honigsbaum, Holmström and Calltorp, 1997). It is partly that the information needed to do so is lacking; partly that the task of comparing the costs and benefits of different services is intrinsically complicated and difficult; and partly that the power structures in the NHS inhibit change even when it is demonstrably desirable. Instead, health service managers responded to the growing pressure on their resources in the latter 1990s in two main ways: by removing some services from the menu of those on offer, and by continuing to allow clinicians the freedom to exercise their own professional judgments in deciding who to treat, and how, within the package of resources that each commands (Redmayne, 1996).

Removing services from the menu of those on offer

A second possible strategy for managing the gap between supply and demand in publicly financed health care systems, which might be regarded as an extreme example of prioritizing, lies in a sharper definition of the range of services that the system provides. Put bluntly, some services that have hitherto been available may be taken off the menu, leaving more resources for the provision of those that remain. It is a process of rationing by exclusion (Klein, Day and Redmayne, 1996), in which those who require the excluded services must either buy them privately or go without.

The best-known and most widely discussed example of rationing by exclusion is the American priority-setting initiative in the State of Oregon, begun in 1994 as a five-year demonstration project (Honigsbaum, Holmström and Calltorp, 1997). The project applied initially only to poor people in the State who were treated under the joint federal and state Medicaid programme, though always with the intention of extending it eventually to small businesses and people with private health insurance. A list is first prepared of all the conditions and their associated treatments that are available under Medicaid, and these 'condition-treatment pairs' are then ranked in terms of their supposed value. Depending upon the amount of money available, a cut-off line is drawn each year across the rankings of the condition-treatment pairs, with none of those falling below it being available to patients under the Medicaid programme. In 1995, 608 out of 744 treatments came above the line and were funded at a level that ensured their availability to all who needed them. Conversely, the 136 treatments falling below the cut-off line were not normally available under the programme.

Although the Oregon project has been widely discussed in the UK, its philosophy has been rejected by successive British governments, which have preferred instead to devolve responsibility for determining priorities to the local health authorities, albeit within guidelines set at the centre. The absence of any official stamp of approval on the policy of rationing by exclusion has not, however, deterred health authorities from quietly dropping certain services from those that are available locally through the NHS. A survey of health authorities' purchasing plans, published in 1995, revealed that 40 of 129 authorities in England and Wales were no longer buying certain treatments (Dean, 1995). They included not only treatments of uncertain value such as the insertion of ear grommets in children and diagnostic dilatation and curettage in women under 40, but also a range of preventive treatments such as the routine use of ultrasound in pregnancy and screening for brittle-bone disease, aortic aneurysm and colorectal cancer. By 1996 almost 70 treatments had been dropped from the NHS by at least one authority in England and Wales, most commonly the reversal of female sterilization, in vitro fertilization, sex change operations, breast augmentation, rhinoplasty, the reversal of male vasectomy, the removal of tattoos, and cosmetic surgery for varicose veins (Klein, Day and Redmayne, 1996, pp. 140–2).

If, as may well be the case, rationing by exclusion is to become more common, the question will increasingly arise of the criteria upon which the exclusions are founded. Experience from the Oregon project confirms the difficulties involved in developing explicit criteria that are both publicly and politically acceptable. There, an iterative series of attempts were made there to rank the large number of condition-treatment pairs in terms of their perceived value. First, they were ranked according to the cost of each treatment and the benefit it yielded; but insufficient data were available to sustain such an approach across all the pairs. Next, they were grouped into 17 categories reflecting the values that the public had been able to articulate through a series of community meetings held throughout the State. The categories included treatments which prevented death, enhanced the quality of life, eased the pain of suffering, and so on. This approach was rejected by the federal government on the ground of possible violation of the statutory rights of disabled people, for many of whom the quality of life was unlikely to improve and who may therefore have suffered under a method giving high priority to treatments judged likely to enhance that quality. Finally, a pragmatic approach was adopted in which priority in the ranking was given to treatments that prevented death, that were less rather than more costly, that emphasized prevention rather than cure, and that eased people's suffering rather than correcting their blemishes.

Although the managers of the Oregon project tried hard to involve the general public in the process of ranking the condition-treatment pairs, the values that emerged from the series of community meetings held throughout the State were inevitably biased towards those who bothered to attend them. A more comprehensively democratic approach to rationing by exclusion has been proposed by Dworkin in his 'prudential insurance principle' (quoted in Smith, 1996a). Like the theories of structural justice that will be considered in Chapter 3, Dworkin's principle is highly abstract and relies upon a number of assumptions that are not replicated in the real world. It may nevertheless provide some valuable insights for those who control the burgeoning process of exclusion. Dworkin invites us to make five core assumptions: that we each have roughly the same levels of income and wealth; that we have full and good information about the effectiveness of different treatments; that we are prepared to act rationally in our own interests; that we value our children's health as much as our own; and that we know nothing about the genetic, cultural or social influences on our health. The government in such an imaginary world would have no reason to be involved in providing health care, since everyone would have the same capacity to insure for the care they needed for themselves and their families. Considerations of equity would not arise. The question that Dworkin invites us to ponder is: which treatments would we choose to be insured for, and which would we regard as not worth the cost of insurance?

Dworkin identifies a number of disparities between the choices that people would probably make in this hypothetical world and the decisions of health care providers in the real world. He suggests, for example, that few people would insure themselves for life-saving treatment if they fell into a persistently vegetative state; yet about 10,000 people are kept alive in such a condition at any time in the US. Few would insure for costly treatment in the last months of an illness that has been diagnosed as terminal, yet some 40 per cent of Medicare expenditure during the last year of life is on people in the last four months of their lives (Lubitz and Riley, 1993). Few, Dworkin suggests, would buy an expensive policy that offered life-saving treatment over the age of 85, though a great deal of such treatment is given at this advanced age. Conversely, most people would insure for immediate and expert treatment for handicapping conditions in childhood, including treatments which are traditionally in short supply such as those for children with speech or learning difficulties.

Dworkin's principle, though restrictive in the assumptions it invites us to make, may offer a genuinely new way of thinking about rationing by exclusion; but it is not one that appears to have influenced the actions of those health authorities in the UK which have been quietly dropping selected treatments from the menu of availability. Certain criteria can, however, be guessed from a simple examination of the discarded treatments (New and Le Grand, 1996). Whether or not a treatment is thought to be effective is an increasingly important element in the scientific evaluation of health care, and therapies of doubtful effectiveness may be at risk. The fairly widespread exclusion of ear grommets and dilatation and curettage may be explained in this way. If cost as well as effectiveness is added into the equation, then other treatments might become candidates for omission, including some expensive drug therapies. Other services, of which in vitro fertilization and a range of cosmetic procedures are relevant examples, may be dropped not because they are ineffective but because they are judged not to form part of the core services that ought to be provided by a publicly funded health service. If people want to achieve assisted fertility or to have their bodies reshaped, then that is a matter for their personal budgets, not for the public purse. Yet other services and treatments may be excluded simply because their demise is unlikely to result in very much political fall-out.

Little of this has reached the stage of public discussion. If anything, the debate in the UK has been the obverse of that in Oregon: not about what might be left off the menu but about what should be included on it. Can we, as Israel has done (Chinitz *et al.*, 1998), identify a core package of services which people are entitled to expect from a modern health care system and which can be guaranteed to be available to all who need them? Agreement about such a package would not eliminate the need for further rationing (unless, of course, the package proved to be extremely small), but it would at least identify the services upon which the rationing debate could focus.

The case in favour of trying to assemble a core package of services for the NHS has been put most clearly by New (1997). He argues that a good deal of health care is special and should therefore be protected in a state-provided package that can guarantee its availability to all who need it. The case rests upon a combination of three characteristics of health care. Firstly, the treatment of people's illnesses and disabilities is fundamentally important, and care should be readily available for every-one whose chances of leading a full and satisfactory life may be put at risk without it. Secondly, since most people have no idea at all about their health care needs over a lifetime, it is unrealistic to expect them to be able to plan for them in the way that they can plan to meet their needs for food, shelter, clothing, education, and even residential care in old age. Thirdly, most people lack the information when they are ill to know either the kind of treatment they require or to judge the quality of the care they are given. Services that embody a major information imbalance of this kind should properly be provided through a publicly funded state-run service rather than the privately financed market-place. The NHS should, New argues, be in the business of providing all the services and treatments which fulfil all the three criteria, and of doing so in a way that guarantees their availability to all who require them. Services that fail to meet the three criteria would be provided only where resources were left over from the core package. Such residual services might include resi-dential care for elderly people, cosmetic dental treatment and medicines for non-complex conditions (New and Le Grand, 1996, p. 53).

So fiercely contested is the arena of health care rationing, however, that for each proposition about a desirable way of proceeding, balancing counter-arguments can be put. While acknowledging the strength of New's case, Klein (1997) questions its practicability. He draws attention, for example, to the difficulties that have been experienced in places which have tried to reach a consensus about a core package of services. It proved impossible in the Oregon project to base the ranking of treatments upon explicit criteria, and resort had finally to be had to the common-sense judgments of the Oregon Health Commission. Similar difficulties have arisen in the Netherlands and Sweden, where the respective governments have declined to specify a basic package of guaranteed care (Sheldon, 1995; McKee and Figueras, 1996). In New Zealand the Core Services Committee, created in 1992 to develop a fair and rational way of determining health care priorities for the nation, was expected to proceed, in the manner of Oregon, by excluding services judged to be of minimal value from the guaranteed core; but this was found to be neither practical nor fair (Honigsbaum, Holmström and Calltorp, 1997, p. 19). Moreover, Klein points out that it has proved extremely difficult in practice for health authorities in the UK to remove even marginally beneficial treatments from the menu. Decisions to close a local service are often met with such a degree of public outrage that the political cost of pursuing the closure becomes too great to bear. In practice, it is only relatively trivial services that have successfully been closed down.

Relying on the courts

A third possible strategy for managing the gap between supply and demand in publicly financed health care systems might be for the courts to seize, or at least to be required to assume, some initiative for determining rules or rights of access to health services in situations where they are in scarce supply. The possibility arises from the fact that the NHS is founded in the statutory will of Parliament. Section 3 of the 1977 National Health Service Act places a duty on the Secretary of State to provide certain specified facilities and services 'to such extent as he considers necessary to meet all reasonable requirements'. Any attempts by the judiciary to become involved in rationing issues of this kind might lie somewhere between first-order and second-order allocations, affecting both the availability of particular services and also their accessibility to particular patients.

For the most part, governments and their agencies in the UK have successfully resisted any legal attempt either to require them to provide a specific volume or standard of care or to guarantee the availability of particular forms of care for those who need them. When the matter has come before them, British courts have usually declined to furnish any such legal guarantees, though recent judgments have shown an apparently increasing appetite by the judges to require health authorities to follow national guidelines. Newdick (1995) has offered a legally informed summary of the current situation:

> . . . these [judgments] give scant encouragement to those thousands of patients whose curable conditions are untreated because beds, wards or entire units are closed for reasons associated with cost. Their effect appears to be that the National Health Service Act creates no direct right to health service resources and that the duty should be considered from the perspective of the various health authorities who must do their reasonable best with scarce resources, subject only to the lightest supervision from the courts. (p. 125)

There have been a number of test cases. One occurred in 1985 when the Court of Appeal considered an application from four patients at a Birmingham hospital who had waited longer than was medically advisable for their treatment (Anon, 1985). The delay had been caused in part by the decision, for reasons of cost, to defer the construction of a new treatment block. The patients sued the Secretary of State, the regional health authority and the area health authority, claiming them to be in breach of the 1977 Act. The Court, however, adhered to the well-established legal principle that ministerial discretion under such a widely framed power could be challenged in the courts only if the decision was so extreme that no reasonable minister could have reached it (Carson, 1987).

In this case, no such extreme behaviour was found, Mr Justice Macpherson pointing out that to decide otherwise would be to lead the country into 'the economics of the bottomless pit'. The health authority's decision was not justiciable. It was for the Secretary of State to decide the extent of services to be provided, and the courts would intervene only if a decision was 'thoroughly unreasonable, irrational, or contrary to the principles of the legislation'. The case left unclear the question of whether the failure to provide treatment in the face of a life-threatening emergency might constitute just such unreasonable or irrational behaviour. The question might have been resolved in 1987 when Angela Tonge threatened to sue the Central Birmingham Health Authority upon being refused renal dialysis for reasons of resource constraints; but litigation was avoided when the Secretary of State suddenly found the wherewithal to provide her with the treatment she needed (Carson, *op. cit.*).

In the much more widely publicized case of Jaymee Bowen eight years later, the Court of Appeal held that the Cambridge Health Authority had not, in fact, acted unlawfully in refusing to fund a specific treatment for a child suffering from an acute life-threatening illness (*The Times Law Report*, 1995). In his judgment the Master of the Rolls, Sir Thomas Bingham, said that difficult and agonizing judgments had to be made about the best ways of using a limited budget to achieve the maximum advantage of the maximum number of patients; but that was properly a matter for the health authorities, not the courts. The Court accepted that in an ideal world every treatment, however slight its chances of success, would be provided; but 'it would be shutting our eyes to the real world if the court were to proceed on the basis that we live in such a world'.

Nevertheless, the removal of specified services or treatments from the menu of those provided by the NHS may be illegal if it manifestly breaches national guidelines. In 1997 the action of the North Derbyshire Health Authority in withholding the supply of Interferon Beta from a patient suffering from multiple sclerosis was held by the High Court to be disingenuous and unlawful (*The Times*, 1997). Mr Justice Dyson ruled that the authority had knowingly failed to apply the national guidance on the use of the drug, which amounted in the view of the Court to an explicit instruction to deny the treatment to patients whom neurologists judged likely to benefit from it. The authority's defence – that it only supported treatments of proven clinical benefit – was set aside. The judgment may increase the difficulties that health authorities will face if, in prioritizing their services, they contravene the growing stream of centrally promulgated guidelines. It remains unlikely, however, that the British courts will wish significantly to influence the management of the gap between supply and demand in the NHS.

Reducing the demand for care

The strategies considered so far that are open to politicians, planners, managers and clinicians in bridging the gap between supply and demand in publicly financed health care systems have a common concern with the total amount of a resource or service that is to be provided. Rationing, in these strategies, is achieved in one way or another through restricting the provision of services. They operate at what Calabresi and Bobbitt (1978) term the first order of allocation. The remaining strategies to be considered are those that influence less the provision of services than the way they are shared out among, and made accessible to, patients. They are strategies that operate more at the second order of allocation.

The next strategy (or, more accurately, assortment of strategies) encompasses a range of activities designed to bear down upon the level of demand for health care. If less use can be made of services, particularly in circumstances that are thought to be inappropriate, resources will be conserved for deployment elsewhere. The mechanisms by which this could be done have been classically summarized by Scrivens (1979). They divide broadly into those that attempt to inhibit demand directly by discouraging patients from entering the health care system in the first place (primary inhibitors) and those that attempt to do so by introducing obstacles that hamper their progress through it once they have got in (secondary inhibitors).

Primary inhibitors

Since access to the NHS for most people is through their GP, primary inhibitors work largely through the family doctor service, seeking to influence people's behaviour even before they enter the doctor's surgery. Put bluntly, they try to stop people from becoming patients. Sometimes they are open and explicit: an example would be the assorted campaigns that have been mounted over the years to educate people about the 'proper' use of their GPs. 'Proper' in the context of such campaigns has meant that people should not trouble their doctors with minor or self-limiting symptoms; they should not call them out at night except in cases of extreme emergency; and they should not expect a prescription at each and every consultation. The introduction of telephone advice help-lines, heralded in the 1997 White Paper, can be seen in part as a further attempt to inhibit the demands made on family doctors by encouraging people to adopt the much less costly alternative of discussing their concerns with a nurse at the end of a telephone line (Pencheon, 1998).

Reception systems in general practice are further examples of primary inhibitors. Knowing how they work from past experience, people may think twice about trying to storm these almost proverbially protective ramparts of primary care. Foster has documented many of what she describes as 'the wide range of informal rationing devices with which GPs can protect themselves against excess demands' (Foster, 1979, p. 492). They include the use of telephone answering services, deputizing services, and the filtering of patients' requests by practice staff. Most commonly used is the appointment system, which by imposing a delay upon access to the doctor or nurse, may discourage some people from trying to get an appointment in the first place and allow others the time for their problems to ease and their appointments to be rescinded.

Less intentionally, there is the fact that, although the NHS is nominally free when people use it, opportunity costs can nevertheless be incurred. Visiting the GP's surgery may involve a financial cost: wages may be lost and transport costs may have to be met. For poor families, such costs can tip the balance between visiting the surgery or staying away. Prescription charges may likewise be an important consideration for people who fall outside the list of exemptions but for whom the cost of one or two prescription items may make the difference between a balanced or a ruined domestic budget for the week.

Secondary inhibitors: delay, denial and dilution

Secondary inhibitors are rather different: they come into play when patients have crossed the threshold of the NHS. In diverse ways they aim to control the demand for care within the system to a level that can be satisfied with the available resources, in much the same way that the sluice gates on a river limit the flow of water to a level that can be contained within the existing banks. The mechanisms that may be involved have been classically identified by Parker (1975). Those most germane to the NHS are delay, denial and dilution, many examples of which will be found in the 'stories' in Chapter 6. Delay may occur in obtaining out-patient appointments to see a consultant and in being admitted as in-patients. Although waiting times are regulated by the Patient's Charter, the number of patients waiting at any moment in time is intractably high, and its reduction has always been seen as a touchstone of the government's commitment to the NHS. At the end of April 1998 more than a million and a quarter patients were waiting to enter NHS hospitals in England, of whom over 47,000 had been waiting for more than a year. Waiting lists can inhibit demand in various ways. Some patients die before they can be admitted, while others get better and are taken off the list: a study of patients waiting for tonsillectomy found that a fifth had grown out of the condition while waiting and were spared the surgeon's scalpel (Freeland and Curley, quoted in Hemingway and Jacobson, 1995). The delay for coronary artery surgery among patients with severe angina must also claim lives before they can reach the operating table.

Denial occurs when doctors and others who control the flow of resources within the system cope with their shortage by the simple device of denying – to their patients and possibly also to themselves – the suitability of a particular treatment or even of any treatment at all. Examples of denial are understandably hard to come by for they touch upon the delicate business of clinical accountability; but the veil was lifted a little by Aaron and Schwartz (1984), whose study of rationing in American and British hospitals was described earlier. Having plotted the extent to which they believed a number of hospital treatments were rationed in the UK, Aaron and Schwartz turned to the intriguing question of how doctors in the UK were able to cope professionally with their role as rationers of care. Many did so, they found, by making the denial of care a matter of routine or even of optimal clinical judgment. Thus, GPs who could not obtain treatment for patients with chronic renal failure explained that nothing could be done other than to make them comfortable. Nephrologists told the families of difficult or troublesome patients that dialysis would be painful and burdensome. Cardiologists restricted the possibility of coronary artery surgery to patients with severe angina, playing down the seriousness of their condition to those with less severe pain.

'In each instance', Aaron and Schwartz commented, 'physicians are asserting that the treatment is *medically* optimal or very close to optimal, and that patients who are denied care . . . because of budget limitations lose essentially nothing of medical significance . . . It enables doctors to avoid the painful realisation that they are doing less than the best for the patient' (*op. cit.*, p. 101). The kind of internal rationalization that takes place was explained by one consultant:

> The sense that I have is that there are many situations where resources are sufficiently short so that there must be decisions made as to who is treated . . . The physician, in order to live with himself and to sleep well at night, has to look at the arguments for not treating a patient. And there are always some . . . In many instances he heightens, sharpens or brings into focus the negative component in order to make himself and the patient comfortable about not going forward. He states the reason for not going forward in medical terms . . . (*op. cit.*, p. 102)

A shortfall of resources has even been proclaimed a virtue: 'at some level we actually need the excuse of limited resources to protect us from the extremes of technological medicine' (Collee, 1995).

Dilution occurs when services are not actually denied but are spread thinly across a greater number of patients, each getting a lesser service than might ideally be the case. Dilution is likely to figure prominently among the informal rationing devices employed by hospitals, the question being not *whether* a particular treatment should be given or a certain procedure carried out, but how comprehensively it should be done. Veatch (1992), for example, has pointed out that, when faced with a clear-cut diagnosis of appendicitis, there is no doubt whatsoever about the value of operating. But that is not the point: the real issue is 'whether to fund countless marginal interventions that are potentially part of the procedure – marginal blood tests and repeat tests, precautionary preventive antibiotic treatment before surgery, the number of nurses in the operating room, and the back-up support on call or in the hospital'. Nor are such marginal decisions confined to the operation itself. Others crop up in the recovery phase: 'how many days of hospital stay are permitted, how often the physician should make the rounds, how many follow up tests there should be, and so on' (quoted in Klein, Day and Redmayne, 1996, p. 113).

Other examples of dilution abound, many of which are illustrated in the 'stories' in Chapter 6. In sub-fertility treatment, the number of menstrual cycles over which the treatment is offered must be decided. In hip surgery a choice has to be made between a titanium prosthesis and a cheaper but less durable steel one. In the treatment of coronary strictures that involve a risk of stroke, a choice must be made between surgery and the cheaper but often less effective alternative of drug therapy. In the treatment of serious leg ulcers a choice can be made between a basic one-layer bandage and a more effective, but also more expensive, four-layer bandage. In many diagnostic pathways a choice must be made about the point beyond which further tests would be possible but costly in relation to the additional information they would yield. And always there is scope for squeezing more work out of over-stretched junior staff (Gilbert, 1998) and for mixing the grades and skills of different professional groups in ways that will allow lesser-paid workers to take on tasks that had previously been done by more costly staff. If the whole spectrum of clinical work were to be dissected in a similar way, the vast scope would become apparent for controlling demand on a day-to-day basis not by the crude bludgeon of denial but the more discriminating rapier of dilution.

Enhancing the efficiency and effectiveness of care

A fifth possible strategy for managing the gap between supply and demand in publicly financed health care systems lies in the imaginatively varied efforts that have been made, and continue to be made, to enhance the efficiency and effectiveness of the health care industry. To walk this road, it is argued, is to generate more beneficial care from a given budget with no diminution in its quality, for it is of the essence of efficiency and effectiveness, in contrast to the devices of delay, denial or dilution, that no compromise needs to be made with standards. And the more beneficial care that can be generated from the budget, the narrower will become the gap between supply and demand and the lesser will be the need for other rationing devices.

Efficiency

Efficiency and effectiveness have been locked in a Siamese embrace at least since Cochrane's seminal essay on them in 1972 (Cochrane, 1972). Efficiency (or, to be more precise, productive efficiency) is about maximizing the quantity and quality of what is achieved from a given quantum of resource. It is about getting the best result for the money available, not getting away with the least amount of expenditure. It can be done in many diverse ways: by ensuring that the right components of care are brought together at the right time in the production process, by buying the needed components at least cost, by ensuring that work is carried out by the least costly staff who are fully competent to do it, by taking advantage of any economies of scale that are available, by eliminating identifiable waste, by maintaining close managerial control over the production process, by investing in research and development to keep abreast of new ideas and appropriate technology, and so on.

The quest for greater efficiency in the NHS has been built into the fabric of the service from the very beginning, and many initiatives have been tried and rejected over the years. They read as a roll-call of the managerial fads and fashions of the service: programme analysis and review, performance indicators, cost improvement programmes, efficiency savings, general management, value-for-money initiatives, Rayner scrutinies, the resource management initiative, clinical budgeting, and others. The 1997 White Paper continued the theme, promising less bureaucracy, a more rigorous approach to performance, and greater incentives to efficiency throughout the service (Department of Health, 1997a). The beneficial effects of greater efficiency on the problem of rationing lie at the heart of the case advanced by the Anti-Rationing Group (Roberts, 1995, 1996). The conclusion appears to be that, preferable though it is to be more rather than less efficient, improved efficiency will neither close the gap between supply and demand nor, therefore, remove the need for other rationing mechanisms to come into play.

The general case for trying to improve the efficiency of the NHS cannot seriously be faulted. To fail to do so is to be reckless in the stewardship of public resources and to incur the charge of corporate mismanagement. Yet the widespread enthusiasm for ever more efficiency must be tempered by the ethical responsibilities of those who manage the service. Staff must not be exploited by paying them less than they merit or causing them undue stress through the imposition of extremely heavy workloads. The quality of the care they provide must not be put at risk through excessively long hours of work. Budgets must not be allowed to be trimmed by shifting an unreasonable or unsupported burden of care onto carers and relatives. Savings in one area of the NHS must not be claimed as a virtue if they have been achieved at the cost of greater expenditure elsewhere. More generally, the truth must not be forgotten that efficiency is to be praised not as an end in itself but only when it is directed towards socially valued purposes. The gas chambers of the concentration camps were doubtless a very efficient way of killing people, but it would be an evil monstrosity to claim such efficiency as meritorious.

Effectiveness

Effectiveness, unlike efficiency, is a notion that is uncontaminated by the pressure of resources and it therefore relates to the problem of rationing in a slightly different way. Treatment A is clinically effective if (to use Cochrane's terminology) it alters the natural history of a disease for the better; and A is more effective than B if it does so more thoroughly, or under a wider range of conditions, or with fewer side-effects. The cost of A and B is immaterial to the question of their effectiveness, though it may be relevant to their affordability. (If, for example, A is not only more effective than B but also more expensive, then a judgement must be made whether it would be a better use of resources to choose B rather than A.) Cochrane's essay startled the medical world on its publication in 1972 with the audacious claim that many treatments currently in widespread use were of no proven effectiveness; but once the shock began to subside, his arguments and ideas became important catalysts in the movement towards the scientific evaluation of medical and surgical treatments. The essential truth of Cochrane's claim has not only become widely accepted in the quarter-century that has since elapsed, it has even been quantified: an informed guess was made in 1991 that only about 15 per cent of medical interventions at that time were supported by solid scientific evidence (Smith, 1991a).

The political and scientific response in the UK to the paucity of evidence about the effectiveness of treatments has been positive. A large amount of research time and money has been committed not only to the scientific evaluation of new and (when ethically allowable) existing treatments but also to the communication of the results, and a number of networks now exist in the UK for the dissemination of the rapidly accumulating body of evidence about therapies that work and the conditions under which they work best. More than that, the introduction of a national scientific programme for research and development in health care in 1991 has ensured that public funds for medical research are channelled where they are judged likely to yield the most handsome dividends in terms of more effective care; and two major centres have been established to provide managers and clinicians with information and advice about the findings emerging from the programme. The 1997 White Paper announced a further raft of initiatives, including a new National Institute of Clinical Excellence to maintain the thrust for what has now come to be called evidence-based medicine (Department of Health, 1997a).

Yet the growing thrust towards an evidence-based style of medical practice may complicate as well as simplify the problem of bridging the gap between supply and demand. Positively, it may highlight the services and treatments which can be dropped from the NHS menu with the least harmful consequences. Yet once the effectiveness of a new drug or treatment has been established, the pressure to make it available to all who might benefit from it will be great, adding to (rather than alleviating) the strains that already exist in health care budgets. The recent discovery of new drugs that appear to be effective in the treatment of Alzheimer's disease, multiple sclerosis, AIDS and impotence are merely compounding the difficulties faced by health authorities in deciding the priority of the items on their shopping lists of services.

Refocusing attention towards prevention

A sixth possible strategy for managing the gap between supply and demand in publicly financed health care systems would entail a readjustment of the balance between the treatment of disease and its prevention. The moderating impact this might have on the problem of rationing is captured in the mythical story of the doctor sitting beside a fast-flowing river. Suddenly, a half-drowned man is swept past in the waters. Instantly the doctor plunges into the river, drags the man to the river bank, and resuscitates him. No sooner has he done so than he sees a half-drowned woman swirling along in the river and he rushes in to rescue her also. And then another man is swept past, and then another woman, and so it goes on until the doctor is brought to the point of exhaustion by his life-saving efforts. As he sits recovering on the river bank, dreading the appearance of yet another person to be saved, he is heard muttering to himself: 'I wish I had the time to go upstream and see who the hell is pushing them in.'

> The pinnacle of achievement in health has come to be equated with the spectacle of men and women becoming over-stressed and under-exercised, indulging in excessive consumption of food, cigarettes and alcohol . . . before being rushed to an intensive care unit and sub-merged in expensive medical technology only when acute symptoms have prevented them from indulging in further consumption. (Draper, Best and Dennis, 1976, p. 28)

The 1990s saw a modest degree of refocusing upstream. *The Health of the Nation* (Department of Health, 1992) and *Our Healthier Nation* (Department of Health, 1998) set ambitious targets for the prevention of disease and premature death and identified wide-ranging strategies for achieving them. Progress towards the targets has been steadier in some cases than in others: death rates from coronary heart disease and from cancer of the breast and cervix have continued to fall, but the prevalence of obesity in adults is rising and there has been little change in the incidence of teenage smoking (Department of Health, 1997b).

Yet although the prevention of disease and the promotion of good health may have been seen by some politicians as a way of limiting the pressure on NHS resources, the true value of prevention is always likely to be intrinsic rather than instrumental. Good health is to be valued for its own sake, not for any easement it might give to the rationing process. It is, in any case, far from clear that improved levels of health in the population will necessarily lead in the long run to lower levels of expenditure on the treatment of disease. In the case of smoking, where the sums have probably been done with the greatest degree of precision, the equation is complex. Fewer smokers will mean less expenditure on the treatment of smoking-related diseases, but such savings will be offset to a greater or lesser degree by a short-term reduction in tobacco revenue and by the long-term survival into old age of cohorts of people who would otherwise have died before their time. Econometric models have generally challenged the widespread belief that smoking imposes a large net burden of cost over time on health care systems (Leu and Schaub, 1983), and the same may be true for other harmful forms of behaviour that yield revenue for the Treasury.

Ethically, too, the arguments surrounding a more pro-active approach to disease prevention and health promotion may be equivocal. There can, of course, be no ethical objection to the policy goal of adding years to life and life to years; but the means by which it is done, and the degree of state power that is brought to bear, may give rise to ethical concerns. If liberty and autonomy mean anything, it must include the liberty to behave in ways that damage one's health. 'It is better to run the risk of cholera and the rest than be bullied into health' thundered *The Times* famously in 1854, rejoicing over the collapse of the local boards of health. The same theme re-emerges in contemporary debates about the moral acceptability of state action to prevent the advertising of cigarettes while it remains legal to sell, buy and use them (Dean, 1991).

Devolving rationing responsibility to clinicians

A final possible strategy for managing the gap between supply and demand in publicly financed health care systems is mediated through the professional autonomy of doctors and other clinicians in their day-to-day contacts with their patients. It reflects the reality that those who most influence the disposition of resources in the NHS are likely to be neither managers nor patients but clinicians – the GPs, for example, through their choices about prescribing and referral, and the consultants through their judgments of whom to treat and how. Through the accumulation of the myriad decisions of daily practice, often taken routinely and without a conscious awareness of the costs they incur, it is the clinicians who largely determine the ways in which the resources of the NHS are rationed among the profusion of patients seeking a share of them. This is, perhaps, micro-rationing in the sense in which it is most commonly understood. It is rationing that is largely hidden and unaccountable, exercised beneath the cloak of clinical discretion, the skirts of which 'society' has not until recently been inclined to lift very far. It is as though there exists an unspoken social contract: 'society' has entrusted to the clinicians the responsibility for taking the ultimate decisions about the allocation of scarce resources, and in return 'society' has absolved the clinicians from explicit democratic accountability for their stewardship of that responsibility.

There is a certain inevitability about the rationing of care through clinical freedom in a publicly funded service where explicit decisions about priorities are avoided or fudged. It corresponds with the realities of the day-to-day work of doctors, nurses and others (as the 'stories' in Chapter 6 attest), and it allows the rationing to be done in flexible and responsive ways. They have already been discussed. Doctors may cope with the gap between supply and demand by delaying the treatment of patients through their management of waiting lists and appointment systems, by denying the suitability or feasibility of treatment, and by spreading the resources more thinly through the dilution of the care they provide. People may sense from their own experiences and those of their friends and relatives that such things go on; and for the most part they allow them to go unchallenged. That is part of the unspoken contract. It is only when an example of, say, explicit denial breaks into the public domain and is magnified by the popular press that the contract creaks at its seams. Such was the case of Jaymee Bowen: although the doctors who were initially responsible for her treatment insisted that their decision to withhold an experimental but possibly life-saving treatment was taken solely in Jaymee's best interests, the media saw it differently (Entwistle *et al.*, 1996). For them, it was a simple case of denying a young child the last chance of life. No matter that the chance was a slim one: it was better than an otherwise certain death, and the doctors who exercised their clinical discretion in refusing to offer the treatment were the subject of a measure of public outrage

The clinical freedom of doctors in the NHS is not, of course, an absolute freedom, nor is it one that absolves them from all accountability for their exercise of it (Hoffenberg, 1987). They are subject to constraints from their profession in the form of standards and codes of conduct; from their colleagues in the shape of medical audit; from their managers in the guise of guidelines and protocols; from their patients in the threat of complaints; and from the courts in the possibility of litigation (Newdick, 1995). Doctors are above neither the law nor the standards of good practice promulgated by their profession, and they must work within both.

In a celebrated editorial in 1983, a senior consultant went so far as to claim that clinical freedom was dead, and that no-one needed to regret its passing (Hampton, 1983). The freedom to which Hampton's paper was an obituary was, however, an old-fashioned freedom exercised by doctors with feet planted firmly in the quicksand of clinical experience. It was the freedom of an earlier era when investigation was non-existent, treatment was as harmless as it was ineffective, and the doctor's opinion was all that there was. That kind of freedom, Hampton argued, 'died accidentally, crushed between the rising cost of new forms of investigation and treatment and the financial limits inevitable in an economy that cannot expand indefinitely'. It should 'have been strangled long ago, for at best it was a cloak for ignorance and at worst an excuse for quackery' (*op. cit.*, p. 1238). Clinical freedom may not be what it was, but it remains alive and well; and signs of its existence are to be seen in the continuing stream of research evidence about widespread variations in the things that doctors do. Klein, Day and Redmayne (1996) seemed to be reflecting a widely assumed view in their assertion that 'despite all the changes in the structure of the NHS, decisions about which patients should be treated, when and how, remain the prerogative of the health care professions' (p. 83).

Intimations of morality

The problems that are set by the seemingly intractable imbalance between the demand for, and supply of, health care in publicly funded systems are many-hued. They are, in part, financial problems: how can the money needed by the NHS best be raised and distributed in the context of a tax-funded service? They are, in part, managerial problems: how is the balance to be decided between the different services offered by the NHS and how can they be provided with the greatest efficiency? They are, in part, clinical problems: how are doctors and other clinicians to decide the order in which patients are to be treated when some must inevitably wait?

They are also, however, moral problems. Little has been written about rationing in the NHS without at least the implicit raising of a moral question about the process. Is the distribution of health care equitable? Are people being treated fairly? How can we justify the discrimination that is an inevitable concomitant of rationing? Are the requirements of social justice being observed? Is the governance of the NHS not only managerially efficient and clinically effective but also ethically defensible?

That such questions are raised at all is interesting, for they are not posed – or not posed with the same degree of insistence – about most other goods and services. We do not usually enquire whether fast cars are distributed equitably or whether people are getting a fair share of designer clothes. It may be a source of envy and covetousness that some people enjoy a cornucopia of luxuries while others go without, but unless the disparities are absurdly wide, we do not usually regard it as *immoral* that wealthier people can have more of them than poorer people. But health care is different. There appears to be something special about health care that marks it out from most, if not quite all, other commodities. Health care seems naturally to attract moral questions in the way that most other commodities do not. Why is this? What is it about health care that is special?

The broad answer given by the literature is that health care is special because of its instrumental power. Health care is the means to an end that is highly valued in western culture: good health and a long life free from pain and disability. Without life-long access to appropriate health care, our chances of attaining this goal may be impaired. Yet the high value that western culture places on good health cannot alone explain the particular status of health care as a focus of moral concern. It is important for us also to have access to food, shelter, clothing, warmth, companionship, mental stimulus, spiritual solace, aesthetic pleasure, love, and other such benefits. Some of these may, for many people, be even more important than a long life or one that is free from pain and disability. What appears to separate health care from the rest is its particular capacity to affect our chances of leading a full, productive and morally fulfilling life. When people experience avoidable ill health and disability, then not only is their enjoyment of life put at risk, so too is their capacity to fulfil the goals they set and the ambitions they nurture. As children they may fail to make the most of their educational potential, handicapping them in the competition for jobs and denying them the status and security that flow from the best of them. As adults, they may be unable to remain in work for any length of time, exposing themselves and their families to the risk of poverty during the working years and on into retirement. As parents, they may be hampered in giving their children the care and support that most parents would wish to do. As citizens, they may feel unable to meet the moral obligations that their country and community expect of them.

It is because of its all-pervading capacity to affect people's chances of succeeding in whatever is important to them in life that the rationing of health care is widely seen as a focus of moral concern. Such a vital commodity must be distributed in a morally acceptable way. People's chances of getting the health care they need cannot be left to the accidents of birth or wealth, ethnicity or gender, whimsy or prejudice. There are, of course, difficulties in this argument, and they will have to be confronted later. For example, not all health care services can be seen by any stretch of the imagination as a vital precondition to a life of fulfilment. Much of what is done in the NHS, in hospitals no less than in general practice, affects the margins of life rather than its centralities. On the other side of the coin, many of the most powerful influences on health lie entirely outside the health care system. Housing, environment, employment, income and genetic inheritance are likely to be as potent predictors of life-chances as the ready availability of good medical care. Nevertheless, the claim has widely been accepted that health care *is* special and that the ways in which it is rationed must be inspected through the prism of moral philosophy; and it is this that the subsequent chapters try to do.

It is, however, unlikely to be the concept of rationing *per se* that attracts our moral attention (Weale, 1990). The need for rationing in health care, in one form or another, could be removed (if at all) only through the allocation of such a large proportion of the national income to health care that any government which tried to do so would rightly stand accused of dereliction of duty. If the job of responsible government is to balance out the nation's varied claims upon the collective purse, then to tip the balance so far in the direction of the NHS that other essential services were grievously damaged would be neither fair nor prudent. It follows, then, that if governments cannot be held to be morally culpable for failing to remove the need for rationing, then rationing itself cannot give rise to legitimate moral concern. And if rationing itself is thus immune from moral attack, so too must be at least some of the mechanisms by which it is done. We cannot allow the principle but condemn all the means by which it is effected. If it is morally acceptable for some people to have to wait for a period of time to receive the care they need, then waiting lists *per se* must also be acceptable (Doyal, 1995). We may wish to look carefully at the way people are moved up and down the lists, but that some must wait seems inescapable.

Further, it can be argued that none of the three main forms of distribution described above (market distributions, rationing by entitlement and rationing by discretion) is *intrinsically* unacceptable on moral grounds. What counts, we may feel, is the way they are allowed to work. Each could operate in morally acceptable ways, and any could work in ways that might arouse our concern. A market distribution, for example, might infringe our sense of justice if the costs of care were always allowed to lie exactly where they fell, without any aid or subsidy for those with the lowest incomes; but it would not do so in a society which, through progressive taxation and redistribution, endowed all of its citizens with an equal purchasing power in the medical market-place. Likewise, rationing by discretion would give rise to no qualms if the discretion were exercised within a set of socially negotiated circumstances under which some patients could justly be preferred over others; but it may do so if those who exercised the discretion were subject to no such constraints over their personal prejudices and preferences. Justice can be delivered in different ways; and so can injustice.

The question, then, is not whether rationing itself is unethical (for it cannot be) or whether particular allocatory mechanisms are unethical (for they cannot be either), but whether they are structured and work in morally acceptable ways and yield morally acceptable results. What are we prepared to accept as a fair basis for discriminating between patients in the rationing process? What arrangement of services is most likely to satisfy our notions of justice and fairness? What do we regard as ethically acceptable ways of making rationing decisions? Are some results of the rationing process more to be preferred, on moral grounds, than others? It is these questions that the next four chapters of the book attempt to address.

2

Choosing between individuals

The issue: a Shavian vignette

George Bernard Shaw may not have been the first to view the ethical dilemmas of rationing through the glasses of an imaginary clinical choice, but the sharpness and clarity of his observation remain a model of perception and wit (Shaw, 1939). In *The Doctor's Dilemma* Sir Colenso Ridgeon, a distinguished physician, has discovered a cure for tuberculosis. 'I have at the hospital', he says, 'ten tuberculosis patients whose lives I believe I can save'. 'Thank God!' responds Mrs Dubedat in relief, for she has come to plead with Ridgeon to treat her husband, an artist, who has the disease. But no more patients can be accommodated, for, as Ridgeon explains, 'my laboratory, my staff, and myself are working at full pressure. We are doing our utmost. The treatment is a new one. It takes time, means and skill; and there is not enough for another case'. 'But how can that be?', objects Mrs Dubedat, 'I don't understand'. 'Try', says Ridgeon, 'to think of those ten patients as ten shipwrecked men on a raft – a raft that is barely large enough to save them – that will not support one more. Another head bobs up through the waves at the side. Another man begs to be taken aboard. He implores the captain of the raft to save him. But the captain can only do that by pushing one of his ten off the raft and drowning him to make room for the newcomer. That is what you are asking me to do'.

Later, as the plot develops, a subtler facet of the dilemma is uncovered. The issue becomes not that of whether one man's life should actually be sacrificed for that of another, but which of two men should be given the one remaining place on the raft. For when Ridgeon decides that he can, after all, accommodate another patient, Dubedat finds he has a competitor for the treatment, Dr Blenkinsop. The two men could scarcely have been cast more differently by Shaw. Louis Dubedat is a young and brilliant artist of great flair and promise, handsome and engaging; but he is also a morally unscrupulous scoundrel. Under false pretences he takes money that he later fails to repay, he borrows valuable artefacts from his acquaintances which he then proceeds to pawn, and he turns out to be an unrepentant bigamist. The elderly Dr Blenkinsop, by contrast, is flabby and shabby, cheaply fed and cheaply clothed. He is one of what Shaw, in his introduction to the play, describes as the hideously poor army of English general practitioners who would be better off financially as a railway porter. In place of an overcoat to protect his consumptive chest, Blenkinsop has to use layers of brown paper. But he is hard-working, diligent and morally upright, doing the best that he can for his patients in deeply unpromising circumstances. He is, moreover, an old colleague of Ridgeon, albeit one who has fallen in his professional life precisely as Ridgeon has risen in his.

To which of the two, Dubedat or Blenkinsop, should Ridgeon offer the only available place in his hospital? The issue is exposed in an exchange between Ridgeon and a fellow physician, Sir Patrick Cullen.

Cullen: Well, Mr Saviour of Lives: which is it to be? That honest, decent man Blenkinsop, or that rotten blackguard of an artist, eh?

Ridgeon: It's not an easy case to judge, is it? Blenkinsop's an honest, decent man; but is he any use? Dubedat's a rotten blackguard; but he's a genuine source of pretty and pleasant and good things.

Cullen: What will he be a source of for that poor innocent wife of his, when she finds him out?

Ridgeon: That's true. Her life will be a hell.

Cullen: And tell me this. Suppose you had this choice put before you: either to go through life and find all the pictures bad but all the men and women good, or to go through life and find all the pictures good and all the men and women rotten. Which would you choose?

Ridgeon: That's a devilishly difficult question . . . It would be simpler if Blenkinsop could paint Dubedat's pictures.

Cullen: It would be simpler if Dubedat had some of Blenkinsop's honesty. The world isn't going to be made simple for you,

> my lad: you must take it as it is. You've to hold the scales
> between Blenkinsop and Dubedat. Hold them fairly.

To put the choice in such a starkly uncompromising way is, to a greater
or lesser degree, to distort reality. Situations may arise in which one life
must be traded off directly against another; but they are probably quite
rare. Yet the need to discriminate among patients when life is not at risk
is a ubiquitous feature of medical practice: clinicians commonly find
themselves having to decide whether to give more care to one patient and
less to another, or more time to this patient and less to that (Gillon,
1985a). As the 'stories' in Chapter 6 reveal, it is part and parcel of their
daily experience. The surgeon who remains in theatre in order to
complete an unexpectedly complicated operation, thereby missing the
scheduled start of his out-patient clinic, is making a choice. So too is the
GP who spends half an hour attending a young woman recently diagnosed with breast cancer and only five minutes seeing a lonely old man
with a sore throat. They are deciding about the right use of their time in
the face of conflicting demands upon it; and, if pressed, they would
presumably have little difficulty in justifying themselves. Their time and
skill, they would say, are best deployed where they are most needed.

Such choices have a moral as well as a clinical dimension to them, for
they invoke the notion of justice. Under what circumstances is it just to
give more time or more care to one patient than to another? The question
is commonly framed in the context of the Aristotelian idea of distributional justice, set out in *Nicomachean Ethics* (Ross, 1966). For Aristotle,
distributional justice – that is, fairness in the way things are shared out
– is not simply a matter of giving people equal burdens and benefits, for
those who will shoulder the burdens and enjoy the benefits are not
themselves equal. It is, rather, about giving them burdens and benefits
that are proportional to relevant differences between them.

The outworking of this beguilingly simple proposition is fraught with
difficulty; but it nevertheless strikes an intuitive cord of agreement. No
elaborate theorizing is needed to justify the GP's decision to spend more
of his time with the woman newly diagnosed as having breast cancer than
with the elderly man and his sore throat. To argue that justice requires
him to spend an equal amount of time with each is patently absurd, for
their situations are palpably different. 'All men agree', writes Aristotle,
'that what is just in distribution must be according to merit in some
sense' (*op. cit.*, p. 112). Those who merit or deserve more should receive
more, and those who merit less should receive less. It is just that the
young woman receives more of her GP's time than the old man because,
in an intuitively correct sense, she merits it. To do otherwise would be

unjust. Stated formally, injustice occurs when 'either equals have or are awarded unequal shares, or unequals equal shares'; and few may quibble with it. As a principle, it feels right and it has stood the test of time.

Yet the main reason for its durability is precisely that it is formal. It is one thing to state, as a formal principle, that unequals should be treated unequally in proportion to their relevant inequalities; it is a different matter to agree the 'relevant inequality' in each particular setting in which the principle is invoked. It is a difficulty that Aristotle anticipated. Having asserted that 'all men agree that what is just in distribution must be according to merit', he goes on to observe that 'men do not all specify the same sort of merit: democrats identify it with the status of freemen; supporters of oligarchy with wealth or noble birth; and supporters of aristocracy with excellence' (*op. cit.*, p. 113). Justifications can usually be found for treating people unequally because of what are claimed to be morally relevant differences between them. Even in the relatively uncomplicated setting of, say, a child's birthday party, some may think that the birthday girl should have a larger share of the cake, since she has in some sense deserved it. 'After all, it is *her* birthday.'

The issue, then, is: on what criteria may people justifiably be treated unequally because they are themselves unequal? What is it about the young woman with cancer that makes her more deserving of her doctor's attention than the old man with a sore throat? In this and many other real-life contexts, the answer is intuitively easier to grasp than it is to explain: the young woman is justified in having a greater share of her doctor's attention because her needs are greater. Having just been told that she has cancer, she needs information, advice, comfort, reassurance and perhaps medication. The old man 'merely' needs someone to talk to and perhaps a linctus to ease his discomfort. It would be difficult to imagine people seriously contesting either the principle that unequal medical needs justify unequal medical treatment or the fact that the woman's medical needs in this particular case are greater than the man's.

Yet moral debate arises most insistently in marginal settings where the principles and the facts are neither readily recognized nor widely agreed. This was the dramatic tension that Shaw created between the gifted but unscrupulous artist Louis Dubedat and the poor but worthy Dr Blenkinsop. Only one can be selected for the treatment of his tuberculosis by Sir Colenso Ridgeon, and while the survival of the chosen one is not guaranteed, the death of the other assuredly is. The choice is a moral one. Values and principles are at stake as well as lives. What is the just or fair allocation of the life-salvaging resource? 'You've to hold the scales between Blenkinsop and Dubedat', says Cullen to Ridgeon. 'Hold them fairly.' But what does 'fair' mean in such a context?

Options for choosing between individuals

Gillon (1985b) finds the outline of an answer in the response of his 8-year-old daughter, Rachel, to a question not dissimilar to that put by Cullen to Ridgeon: how should one out of three dying people be chosen to have the only available life-saving machine?

> 'Well', she told me, sparing a minute or two from her television programme, 'you could give it to the illest because she needs it most, or you could give it to the youngest because she'd live longer, or you could give it to the kindest because kind people deserve to be treated nicely. No, you couldn't give it to the one you liked best, that wouldn't be fair.' Nor, she decided, would 'eenie meenie minee mo' be fair because the one who needed it most, or the youngest, or the kindest might not get it. Nor did she (much to my surprise) think that the Queen should get it in preference to the poor man 'because she's got so much already and the poor man hasn't.' Of all the methods, her preferred one was to choose the illest because she needed it most – but, not surprisingly, she could not say why that was a better option than the others. (*op. cit.*, p. 267)

Here is a delightful summary of what are probably the main criteria which could be invoked in preferring either Louis Dubedat or Dr Blenkinsop for treatment by Sir Colenso Ridgeon.

Need

Needs and wants

Of Rachel Gillon's several possible criteria for justifying the preferential treatment of one patient over another, her first, that of need, is probably the most widely understood and accepted. People who are ill need treatment, and those who are most ill need it most. Health care addresses some of the most fundamental needs of human beings, and all else being equal, the greater the need the more potent the moral claim on the resources of the health care system. If illness threatens people's capacity to flourish as human beings and to attain the goals and satisfactions they seek, then the greater the threat, the greater the need and the more insistent the moral claim to preferential treatment. It is this which sustains the high priority that is given to life-saving treatments, both in theory and in practice, for there is no greater threat to the attainment of goals and satisfactions than the imminence of avoidable death.

Although the idea of 'need' has commonly been seen as the single most important basis for the morally acceptable distribution of health care services, it has proved to be almost as difficult to handle in practice as it has been attractive in theory. One difficulty lies in the very definition of need, for people's needs can all too easily transform themselves into wants, the satisfaction of which may be more a matter of economics than of morality. Circumstances can, of course, be imagined in which the distinction is perfectly clear. If I require an operation to save my life, then I may rightly be seen as having a moral claim on the resources that are necessary to carry it out, for otherwise my capacity to flourish as a human being is placed at very grave risk. Under any definition, I both want and need the operation. Yet I cannot say with the same degree of conviction that I need designer clothes or a fast car. I may *want* them, perhaps very badly. I may even be willing to pay the asking price for them. But it would be stretching the normal use of language to claim that I need them in quite the same way that I need an operation when my life is threatened. Things that are needed to maintain the integrity of a flourishing human life are morally different from those that are simply wanted or desired (Doyal and Gough, 1991).

Yet beneath this surface of common understanding the distinction between needs and wants is a slippery one, not least in the context of health care. On the one hand, by no means all forms of health care are concerned with needs that would be damaging to human flourishing if left unmet. As much as a third of all the illnesses seen by general practitioners will probably improve of their own accord, whether or not they are treated, and even a good deal of surgery is aimed at enhancing people's comfort or appearance rather than saving their lives or enhancing their capacities. Is such care to be regarded as meeting a fundamental human need? On the other hand, the intensity of certain wants can be such that the failure to satisfy them may cause deep psychological or other harm. Women who perceive their breasts to be either much too large or much too small may be driven to the edge of despair by their negative self-image even though breast size *per se* is not usually a medical condition requiring treatment. The notion of want may then slide imperceptibly into that of need, blurring an otherwise clear distinction between them.

The difficulty of separating needs from wants has to some extent been resolved in the literature through the distinction between subjective and objective judgments of need. Subjective needs are those which people define themselves as having. To say that 'I am desperate for a cigarette' or, to use the language of mortal risk, that 'I am dying for a drink' is to express not only a perfectly valid sense of what I wish to have, but also the urgency that I attach to having it. It is, however, just that – what *I* think I need. Others may disagree, and in the case of cigarette smoking they probably will. What I need, they may aver, is not a cigarette but access to the kind of help that will enable me to kick the habit. They would not agree that my own assessment of my psychic state as one of need would give me any moral claim to a cigarette or a drink, and certainly not at public expense!

To externalize or objectify the judgment of need is helpful in escaping the difficulty that wants and needs can all too easily shade into one another. What may matter, at least for the purpose of moral judgment, is not what I consider myself to need but what others believe me to need. Merely to have one's need adjudged by someone else is not, however, itself sufficient to justify a moral claim. Topers engaged together in their favoured pastime may readily adjudge each other to need another drink. What seems to count is not only the external judgment itself but also the authority on which it rests. Topers have not a shred of moral authority to pronounce upon the beverages needed by others. From this point of view, needs are valid only if they are endorsed by people who are in some way sanctioned or licensed for the task (Bradshaw, 1972). In western societies it is doctors who are allowed to adjudicate a patient's need for medical care and it is they who can articulate the consequences of a patient's failure to receive such care. Doctors have this power not because they have abrogated it to themselves in the face of opposition from the people, but because the people, through the socially negotiated mechanisms that register and regulate the doctors, have allowed them to acquire and exercise it.

Relative need and medical triage

This particular difficulty does not arise in the case of Dubedat and Blenkinsop, for each has a life-saving need for Ridgeon's treatment. Ridgeon himself, a legally registered doctor, has confirmed this to be the case. Dubedat and Blenkinsop do not merely want the treatment that Ridgeon can offer, they need it. Rather, the issue in their case is whether the need of one is greater than that of the other. Rachel Gillon's view was that, in choosing between three people for the one place on the life-saving machine, the illest could justifiably have priority because 'she needs it most'.

Such a view chimes in with common sense. There are, self-evidently, needs and there are needs. Judging from the rate at which cough medicines and nasal drops are prescribed, doctors habitually identify a great deal of need among patients with upper respiratory infections; but such needs can hardly compare with the needs of those suffering from, say, cancer, nephrotic kidneys or motor neurone disease. But how are they to be separated out? How can it be ascertained whether this person's need is greater than that person's, justifying his or her priority claim on scarce resources?

The problem may be more one of theory than of practice, for the notion of medical triage has long been found to be a practicable way of grading the severity of patients' needs for health care and determining the order in which they should be treated (Winslow, 1982). Triage, which derives from an obsolete meaning of the verb 'to try' – to separate – has come to acquire the meaning of sorting or grading objects according to their quality (*Oxford English Dictionary*). In the early eighteenth century, triage was used to describe the actions of wool merchants in separating fleeces according to the firmness of the wool, and the term was later applied to the action of coffee harvesters in grading the quality of the beans they were picking. Coffee made from the worst beans was known as 'triage coffee'.

By the early twentieth century, triage had become confined almost exclusively to the medical domain, particularly in contexts of war where rapid decisions had to be made under battle conditions about the order in which wounded personnel would be treated in field hospitals. The triage nurse or doctor was the one who prioritized the cases, sometimes on the basis of the severity of the injuries, sometimes on the speed at which the wounded could be patched up and returned to action. Later, the term was taken into the language of the civilian hospital, and hospital accident and emergency departments now commonly adopt a form of triage in which the condition of each new admission is speedily assessed by a triage nurse and people are treated in the order of their clinical severity.

There is, however, an important distinction between military and civilian triage. Triage in the theatre of war may give priority in treatment less to those whose injuries are clinically the most severe than to those who can be returned most quickly to the front – and these may, paradoxically, be the least severely injured. Where this happens, triage functions to maximize a corporate advantage, not to meet the most pressing of individual needs. It is more important under battle conditions to maintain the fighting capacity of the army than it is to treat those in greatest clinical need. In World War II, for example, scarce supplies of penicillin in the US army were used in the treatment of venereal disease in preference to that of infected wounds, for it was in this way that soldiers could be returned more quickly to the front

(Beauchamp and Childress, 1989, p. 299). The collective benefit to the social group may or may not be a morally relevant criterion justifying a priority claim on resources. It trespasses into the territory of utilitarianism, which is the subject of Chapter 5. Suffice it here to note that the capacity to benefit from treatment is not the same as the severity of the needs of individual patients.

Similar issues may arise also in civilian contexts. Shaw tells us nothing of the clinical histories of Dubedat and Blenkinsop other than that each has tuberculosis; but suppose that one of them also has an additional life-threatening disease. Since the combination of the two diseases might pose an even graver risk to life than tuberculosis alone, the one who was suffering this double catastrophe might be said to have, in some qualitative sense, a greater need than the other because the threat to his 'flourishing' would be that much greater. It would follow, then, that he should have the prior claim on resources since his would be the greater need. At the very least it would be doubly unfair to discriminate against him simply because of his extra morbidity. Yet precisely because his prospect of survival was the lesser of the two, the case might be made that the finite quantum of care should be given to the one with the better chance of survival – the one, that is to say, with the lesser but still grave need. To argue in this way is again to substitute need as the criterion of choice with some notion of social accounting in which the best return is obtained for the resources expended. It is utilitarianism in another guise.

The diaspora of need

The cases of Dubedat and Blenkinsop, as presented by Shaw, do not involve a judgment about the *relative* need of each man. Each has tuberculosis and each may die unless treated. Their personal needs are equal, and that is all we know about their clinical conditions. Yet there could be a sense in which, even when faced with an apparently equal personal need for treatment, the notion of relative need could be properly invoked. Suppose that one of them has dependent children, and the other does not. The balance of need may now be thought to have shifted. It is no longer simply a matter of whether one should receive the treatment and live, but of whether the 'flourishing' of several individuals is to be weighed against that of a single person – for we may assume that the children would suffer if it were their father who was passed over for treatment and died. Need becomes dispersed, a diaspora, not just a personal quality.

From this perspective, the needs of the two contenders for treatment would not be equal – far from it. There is evidence, moreover, that such a perspective is not just an imagined one: the so-called God-Committees which meet to determine the allocation of patients to renal dialysis programmes often take account, among many other things, of the family dependants of each patient under consideration (Calabresi and Bobbit, 1978, pp. 187–8). The question may be asked, though, where the boundaries of the diaspora of need might end. If need can extend to dependent children, why not also to other dependent relatives, or dependent employees, or dependent colleagues? To pose the question is to move farther away from the notion of personal need as a morally relevant criterion towards other criteria (such as social or economic worth) that merit separate consideration.

Age

The criterion of need, crucial though it may be in other contexts, is of little help in resolving the choice between Dubedat and Blenkinsop. Each has a need for Ridgeon's treatment, and each one's need, moreover, is absolute. If either man does not receive the treatment he will die. The next criterion enunciated by Rachel Gillon, that of age, is however of much more obvious relevance: 'you could give it to the youngest because she'd live longer'. Dubedat, we are told, is only 23 years of age. Blenkinsop, by contrast, is a much older man: although his precise age is not revealed, he is a near-contemporary of the fifty-ish Sir Colenso.

The principal argument about the moral relevance of age in the selection of patients for treatment is that of the fair innings (Harris, 1985). All else being equal, younger people should have priority over older people simply because they have had less chance of achieving whatever it is they wish to achieve in life. To treat an older person, thereby letting a younger one die, would be inherently unjust in terms of each one's years of life. The younger person would get no more years than the relatively few she has already had, while the older person would add several more to the many she has already enjoyed.

Reasons can be adduced both for and against the proposition. In its favour is its appeal to altruism and even to common sense: all else being equal, it seems self-evidently fair that, say, a 20-year-old should have priority over a 70-year-old if their claims come into conflict. What possible grounds could there be, in equity, for preferring the older of the two? In what sense would it be fair to give a small extension of life to an older person at the cost of a large extension to a younger one? It is a powerful case that appears to be accepted not only in daily clinical practice (Dean, 1994) but also in formal guidelines. In New Zealand, for example, patients over the age of 75 with kidney failure are not usually considered for dialysis or transplantation (Honigsbaum, Holmström and Calltorp, 1997, p. 27). Central to the case, however, is the notion of the life-span: what counts is the chance that each person has to flourish across a normal span of life, not at any particular age. The argument favours the young over the old not because the 20-year-old has an intrinsically stronger claim than the 70-year-old but because their prospects over the course of a normal life-span should be made as equal as possible.

It is precisely this that is challenged by those who reject age as a morally relevant criterion. Grimley Evans (1997), for example, argues that people of all ages have a right to be treated as individuals, not as uniform members of a class, whether that class is based on sex, skin colour, wealth or age. Older people are just as heterogeneous as younger ones, and while it is true that older people *as a group* have a lesser expectation of life than younger people, it may not be true of older *individuals.* People age, biologically, at very different rates (Grimley Evans, 1995), and to treat each individual according to a group stereotype is a blatant case of ageism. It is unfair to discriminate against someone who is not responsible for the variable on which the discrimination is based and who may already be experiencing a reduction in health and vitality. In any case, as the geriatrician's 'story' in Chapter 6 attests, medical care of the elderly is now so good that many conditions of old age, for which treatment might formerly have been a waste of money, can be treated successfully. Who is to say that an extra ten years of life at an older age will not be productive of as much happiness and fulfilment as 30 years at a younger age?

Such arguments, other than in their most extreme form, do not claim that older people should *never* come out second best in the competition for care, merely that their age is an irrelevance in the choice. Other, more morally appropriate criteria might in some cases work in favour of older people and in some cases against them; but the choice should be based on those alternative criteria and not pre-empted by the irrelevance of age. A similar position appears to have been adopted by the British Medical Association, whose spokesman on ethics was reported in 1998 to have described it as ethically dubious that 'doctors are making blanket policies about treating patients . . . They should all be treated as individuals, not on the basis of some classification' (quoted in Johnston, Calvert and Connett, 1998). To the extent that public opinion can be gauged through interviews and surveys, however, people generally appear to approve of the notion of the 'fair innings'. Half of the respondents in a national survey in 1995 agreed that higher priority should be given to the treatment of the young than the elderly, and respondents in a Gallup survey accorded priority to small babies, those with family responsibilities, and previously healthy young and middle-aged people (Kneeshaw, 1997). By invoking the preferences of the people, Mrs Dubedat might be strengthened in her pleas for her husband.

Personal merit

The same may not be true, however, were she to rely upon the next criterion enunciated by Rachel Gillon, that of personal merit. 'You could give it to the kindest because kind people deserve to be treated nicely.' The issue was put to Sir Colenso Ridgeon, quite brutally, by Sir Patrick Cullen. 'Well, Mr Saviour of Lives: which is it to be? That honest, decent man Blenkinsop, or that rotten blackguard of an artist, eh?' Ridgeon's immediate response may strike us as oddly equivocal: 'It's not an easy case to judge, is it?' To most people, perhaps, it is very easy indeed to judge: personal traits such as honesty and trustworthiness are simply irrelevant in determining the just distribution of scarce resources for medical care. So too are the obverse traits of mendacity, greed, and so forth. To allow their relevance would, many might argue, be to open a particularly difficult and offensive can of worms, reminiscent of earlier categorizations of the deserving and undeserving poor.

First, there would be the problem of agreeing which of a large number of personal traits to allow. If honesty and niceness can justify preferential treatment, why not thrift, charity, courage, fortitude, chastity, and other traditional virtues? Next, there would be the problem of defining them. What, precisely, are the particular hallmarks of niceness and kindness? How charitable does one have to be in order to be counted charitable? How thrifty to be counted thrifty? And it can easily be imagined how impossible it would be to quantify the amount of each relevant virtue among a large number of people in a way that would enable them to be compared reliably and fairly. The public guardians of civil liberties would doubtless have much to say about any attempts to do so.

But none of these practical difficulties gets to the heart of the matter: whatever the feasibility of the proposition, is it morally right to distribute scarce and valued public resources on such a basis? And if it is not, why not? At least two different kinds of answer may be given. The first is that, if the moral relevance of personal virtue is conceded, other more valued criteria may be overruled. People's needs for care, however problematic their definition and measurement, appear to be much stronger grounds for claiming priority in treatment; and to allow need to be trumped by personal virtue would be to deny the weight that we might wish to give it. The primary moral obligation when faced with someone in need is to offer help appropriate to their condition, not to enquire about their virtues.

An alternative answer relies upon the slippery notions of free will and responsibility. The case for treating nice people preferentially rests upon the assumption that they have, in some sense, deserved the advantage. Their niceness or kindness is a result of their own efforts, and their preferential treatment is a just reward for their diligence. Conversely, those who are nasty or cruel are assumed to be responsible for their negative traits and can thus be fairly penalized for them. In reality, the links between free will, responsibility and personality are in all probability much more complex than this simple assumption allows. Traits and dispositions are forged over long periods of time from diverse inheritances and experiences, some of which may be much more volitional than others. To argue, simply, that nice people are what they are because of the personal virtues which they have volitionally nurtured is to distort the reality of human development to an unacceptable degree.

None of this would matter if personal merit or fault were never used as a basis for discrimination, either positively or negatively, in the selection of patients for treatment. Yet there is a particular circumstance in which it could occur, namely where people's health care needs are held to result from their own reckless behaviour, and treatment is accordingly withheld. Patients then become the victims of a double jeopardy: not only is their health impaired by their behaviour, they are also discriminated against for treatment because their condition is seen to be, in some sense, their 'own fault'.

In 1993 Harry Elphick, a 47-year-old smoker, was refused cardiac surgery when he was admitted to Wythenshawe Hospital in Manchester following a heart attack (*The Times*, 1993). He might have benefited from surgery on his coronary arteries, but the initial X-ray examination of the arteries (angiography) was not usually given to regular smokers referred to the hospital. Since his condition was not judged by the cardiologists to be urgent, Mr Elphick was advised to enrol in a smoke-stop clinic prior to being reassessed for treatment at a later time. The advice was accepted, and through the help of his GP Mr Elphick successfully gave up smoking; but before he could be reassessed by the hospital he suffered a further heart attack and died.

The case of Mr Elphick was widely seen as one of blaming the victim, as was also the later one of Michelle Paul who was allegedly denied a liver transplant on the grounds that she had caused her own crisis through the misuse of drugs (Bowditch, 1997). The cardiology department, hard pressed to keep within its operating budget, was represented in the media as having made a moralistic judgment to withhold treatment from Mr Elphick because he had brought the condition upon himself. The medical staff, however, insisted that their decision to withhold treatment was motivated neither by a moralistic condemnation of his smoking nor by a conscious weighing of the opportunity costs of treating him. Rather, they contended, it was a straightforward clinical decision based solely on what they regarded to be in his best interest. Not considering his life to be in danger, they judged that he would best be treated first by inducing him to stop smoking and then by offering him surgical or medical intervention as appropriate. To operate while he was still a smoker would be to run a higher risk of death during the operation and to require more time on a ventilator after it. Far from rejecting him, the doctors insisted that they were actually treating him in the best possible way, beginning with the preliminary phase of eliminating the harmful constituents of tobacco from his blood stream. This explanation must, of course, be accepted. Yet the case of Mr Elphick raised the important question of whether such a stance would in principle be ethically permissible. Is a self-induced condition a morally relevant criterion for withholding or modifying treatment in circumstances where choices have to be made?

Instinctively, the answer appears to be 'no', and for much the same reasons that niceness and kindness strike us as inappropriate reasons for the positive selection of patients. As a purely practical consideration, where would it end? If patients needing treatment for smoking-related diseases can fairly be penalized because they smoke, why not apply the same stricture to those who drink too much alcohol, eat too much fat, drive too fast a car, work too hard, or indulge themselves in dangerous sports? Few of us, on such a basis, might qualify for the treatment we required in our hour of need. And is it fair to assume that such behaviour is indeed volitional – for it is upon this assumption that the argument appears to hinge? Nicotine is now widely recognized (even by the cigarette manufacturers) as a potently addictive drug, and alcoholism and eating disorders are diseases in their own right. At the very least, the proposition that we have volitionally brought many of our ills upon ourselves must be challenged and tested in each situation in which it is invoked.

More important even than these considerations is the moral obligation of the clinical professions to offer appropriate care whatever the cause of a patient's condition. There is nothing in the traditional codes of medical practice exempting doctors from the care of patients who happen to be the victims of their own intemperance (see Chapter 4). Quite the reverse: ethical opinion now regards it as explicitly impermissible for doctors to be biased in their decisions by any knowledge they may possess about the causes of their patients' ills. In the wake of public concern about the case of Mr Elphick, the British Cardiac Society explicitly dissociated itself from any clinical policy that 'systematically denies the right of access to treatment . . . on the basis of specific risk factor, *even if this is self-induced*' (quoted in Hughes and Griffiths, 1996, emphasis added). Two years later, in a booklet of ethical guidance published in 1995, doctors were forbidden by the General Medical Council to refuse the treatment of patients with unhealthy habits. The President of the Council was quoted as saying: 'A doctor cannot insert his own view of a patient's lifestyle and . . . punish the patient by withholding treatment for, say, smoking' (*The Times*, 1995). It is a view that reflects a long tradition of altruism. Before ministering to his needs, the Good Samaritan did not enquire about the mugged man's prudence in venturing alone along a notoriously robber-infested route.

Nevertheless, the matter may appear in a different light to those who feel themselves to be the losers in such circumstances. Non-smokers can often obtain life-related insurance cover at lower rates than smokers, and few would regard this as a cause for moral concern. Why should non-smokers not also have the advantage in the competition for scarce public resources? If I who have never smoked were to receive inferior treatment for my blocked arteries than my neighbour who is a life-long smoker (which might happen if the fact of his smoking is held to be irrelevant and the choice of our treatment is made on other grounds), I might feel myself to have been unfairly treated. Righteousness, even if it is endowed through our genes rather than won by our virtue, may still be thought to count for something by those who possess it.

Personal appeal

If the personal merit of the patient is a contestable criterion in the fair allocation of resources, even more so is likely to be the next option identified by Rachel Gillon: his or her personal appeal to the doctor. You could, she said, give it to the one you liked the best. For doctors to allow their personal feelings for their patients to cloud their behaviour towards them is, at its most extreme, indubitably unethical. Herein, it finally transpires, lies Sir Colenso Ridgeon's nemesis, for it was finding himself hopelessly in love with Dubedat's wife, Jennifer, that led him to relinquish his care of the artist to Sir Ralph Bloomfield Bonnington, believing (correctly, as it happened) that Dubedat would die.

Ridgeon: Something has got me by the throat: the truth must come
        out. I used the medicine myself on Blenkinsop. It did not

	make him worse. It is a dangerous medicine: it cured Blenkinsop: it killed Louis Dubedat. When I handle it, it cures. When another man handles it, it kills – sometimes.
Jennifer:	Then why did you let Sir Ralph give it to Louis?
Ridgeon:	I'm going to tell you. I did it because I was in love with you.
Jennifer:	You tell me that! To my face! Callously! You are not afraid!
Ridgeon:	I am a doctor. I have nothing to fear.

Ridgeon should, of course, have a great deal to fear. Deliberately to put the life of a patient at risk because of a lust for his wife is among the blackest crimes in the professional book. Few, if any, would condone it and few would view it as a morally acceptable solution to the doctor's dilemma. The prophet Nathan had some harsh words for King David when he used his regal power to engineer the death of the cuckolded Uriah in order to marry his widow, the pregnant Bathsheba; and so too should the General Medical Council for Sir Colenso.

At a much less malign level, however, is the natural human experience of finding oneself in greater sympathy with some people than others and more favourably disposed towards them in our dealings with them. The 'teacher's favourite' is to be found not only in the classroom but on the shop floor, in the office, on the parade ground, and in the surgery. Of course, a certain sympathy, or quality of imagination, is a potent weapon in the doctor's armoury (Limentani, 1997). It enables the physician to enter, in his imagination, into the lives of his patients; to see their world in some measure as they see it; and to tailor his approach to their problems in ways that resonate with their own outlook and under-standing (Berger and Mohr, 1967). Yet unless carefully constrained within the boundaries of professional propriety, sympathy may all too easily transmute into something less laudable. From sympathizing, in a professional sense, may come liking; from liking may come the desire to please; and from the desire to please may come the unconscious exercise of preference and bias. Whatever may be their formal professions of detached neutrality, doctors do respond differently to patients with whose conditions they can sympathize (Griffiths and Hughes, 1994). And the reverse may also be true: scattered throughout the literature on medical practice are the 'heartsink' patients – those who repeatedly appear with imagined or intractable symptoms and who may be dis-missed with less courtesy or care than others who are grateful or clinically interesting. 'There are', O'Dowd (1988) has written, 'patients in every practice who give the doctor . . . a feeling of "heartsink" every time they consult. They evoke an overwhelming mixture of exasperation, defeat and sometimes plain dislike that causes the heart to sink when they consult' (p. 528).

Understandable and perhaps even unavoidable though the existence of such sentiments might be, we are offended by the idea that they might influence the selection of patients for care in situations where choices have to be made. Rachel Gillon was clear about this: 'you couldn't give it to the one you liked best, that wouldn't be fair'. Personal appeal, even of a much more honourable kind than Jennifer aroused in Ridgeon, may conflict with other, stronger principles such as need or benefit, and it may open the door to corruption, bribery and prejudice. It may erode trust, foster secrecy in the disposition of public funds, and lack accountability. It is, we may presume, not to be commended as a morally relevant quality. And yet, as the 'stories' in Chapter 6 reveal, heartsink patients can become conveniently lost in the backwaters of a waiting list.

Social esteem

The last substantive criterion cited by Rachel Gillon for determining who among a small number of contenders should have the last remaining place on a life-saving machine is that of social esteem. You could, she said, prefer the Queen to the poor man. The notion of social esteem is close to that of personal merit and might perhaps best be seen as a variant of it. A distinction may, however, be made between them. Personal merit is concerned with *what* we are; social esteem is concerned with *who* we are. The Queen may be a thoroughly nice person; but that is not the point. In the context upon which Rachel Gillon was pronouncing, the Queen's privilege, if it is conceded, would be based upon her position, not her personal qualities. It would derive from the esteem accorded to her as the head of state, irrespective of her personal merits or failings.

To choose the monarch as the exemplar of social esteem is, to a degree, misleading. It is to be expected that a head of state will have access to a private or privileged source of health care, and few may quibble about it. When Queen Elizabeth the Queen Mother underwent a successful hip replacement operation on the same day in 1995 that an independent survey revealed that one in three health authorities had introduced explicit rationing, little fuss was made in the media of the large number of her less privileged subjects waiting in pain for their own operations (Dean, 1995). To have done so would have been inappropriate for all but the most zealous egalitarian. But as we descend the hierarchy of social esteem, doubts may accumulate about its moral relevance in the allocation of health care.

Early in 1983 a 42-year-old man came under the care of the renal unit at the Churchill Hospital in Oxford (Brahams, 1985). He had a history of psychiatric illness, hypertension, impaired renal function and severe mental impairment. He lived, when fit enough, in a protective hostel for the homeless. As time went by his renal function worsened to the point where dialysis was required. As soon as dialysis began, in March 1984, the man's mental state deteriorated and other medical problems also emerged. Extensive areas of cerebral damage were found, with cortical loss consistent with infarction. The patient became demented and his mental age was put at about three. He did not respond to simple questions; he was at times violently unco-operative; he was incontinent of urine and faeces; he could not take his medication reliably; and he exposed himself and masturbated while being examined.

After a period of time in which the dialysis sessions became an increasing torment to both the patient and his nurses, the decision was finally taken by the renal unit in December 1984 to discontinue his treatment. Because of their expected fierce opposition to the decision, neither the patient's GP nor the staff of the hostel in which he was living were consulted. On learning of it they protested, claiming that he had a reasonable quality of life; and although the hostel staff offered to accompany him on future visits to the unit, the offer was declined. A reassessment of the case was made by the area medical officer, but the decision to discontinue treatment was upheld. Following pressure and financial aid from the British Kidney Patient Association, the man was dialysed for a time in a private unit and plans were drawn up for the installation of a dialysis unit in the hostel; but he died in April 1985.

The case has several strands, only one of which touches upon the question of social esteem. It was widely seen at the time to be an exceptional case since it hinged not around the text-book dilemma of whether to offer dialysis to a new patient who has not yet begun the treatment but whether to discontinue it for one who is already receiving it. It was observed that, although a shortage of resources was not a dominant factor in the case, a fair and sensible allocation of the unit's resources had to be taken into account (Brahams, 1985). By implication, it was judged to be fair and sensible to withdraw dialysis from this particular patient. Why? The renal team was reportedly of the view that continuing dialysis would no longer be in his best interest. His medical condition was poor and deteriorating. Yet that scarcely seems to be a *general* justification for withdrawing a life-preserving treatment, and in any case the man was apparently able to function tolerably well within the protected boundaries of the hostel. There must be at least the suspicion that the choice reflected the view of the renal team that his life was to all intents and purposes socially worthless. He represented almost nothing of what is socially esteemed in modern Britain. Had the life in question been that of, say, a 42-year-old businessman or schoolteacher, with similar compounding medical complications, would the same decision have been taken?

To put the question in this way is, however, to shift the terms of the debate somewhat away from the 'pure' notion of social esteem to the rather more 'applied' notion of social contribution. The businessman or the schoolteacher may indeed be preferred to an awkward homeless man not only because they enjoy a greater esteem in the eyes of society but also because their past and (possibly) future contributions to the common good are that much the greater. It is this facet of the notion of esteem that Shaw exploited in *The Doctor's Dilemma*, where he made the choice to lie between Dubedat, the uniquely talented creator of beautiful things, and Blenkinsop, the workaday doctor whose craft could be replicated by a large army of medical foot-soldiers. It was not a question of whether the one enjoyed a greater status or prestige than the other but of which of the two had contributed the more to human happiness – and which had the greater potential to do so in the future? Sir Patrick Cullen puts the point thus: 'To me, it's a plain choice between a man and a lot of pictures'. To which Sir Colenso Ridgeon replies: 'It's easier to replace a dead man than a good picture'.

Rachel Gillon was clear that social esteem, at least in its 'pure' form, cannot be a morally relevant ground for distinguishing between people's claims for health care. Quite the reverse: she favoured the mirror principle of social compensation. The Queen has 'got so much already and the poor man hasn't'. Far from being a reason for passing people over, their low social esteem becomes, from this perspective, a relevant criterion that actually justifies their preferential treatment. It is not a matter of who people are or what they have contributed to society but of what society can do to them to compensate for their misfortunes. To each according to their need, not their status.

The case may strike us as a good one; though if it does, we have to explain why we might be prepared to make an exception in the case of the Queen Mother. That apart, it does seem unfair that some people should be penalized simply because they are thought to be of lesser social esteem than others or because they have less to give to the common good. To do so might, in practice, be to allow certain groups of people to become the victims of systematic disadvantage. It would compound our feeling of injustice if the grounds for determining the low social worth of people's lives were those over which they had little volitional control. It is the argument of free will and responsibility appearing again under a slightly different guise. If (though of course we cannot know) the man who was taken off the dialysis programme at the Churchill Hospital in 1984 was nothing more than the hapless victim of an accumulation of genetic and experiential misfortunes over which he had had little if any personal control, then to deprive him of continuing life on the ground that that life was of negligible esteem or worth was to compound his unmerited misfortune. He was not, in any reasonable sense, responsible for the dreadful predicament in which he found himself, and it was unjust that it should be held against him. Rather, as Rachel Gillon seems to argue, he should have been the recipient of supererogatory care since he had so little else going for him.

It may, on the other hand, be argued that, if all else is equal, the contribution that people make to the well-being of their society is indeed a proper factor to be taken into consideration. What would be so terribly unfair about choosing the singularly talented artist in preference to the reproducible artisan when all else between them is equal? Or the Nobel prize winner rather than the dull teacher? It may be bad luck that none bar the very few has a sublime artistic or scientific talent – but that's life. Justice does not require us to refrain from discriminating among people *at all*, merely to refrain from doing so on the basis of morally irrelevant criteria. In what sense, then, could the skills and talents of those who can contribute most to the common good be regarded as irrelevant? Does not the very fact of their potential for communal benefit endow them with a shimmering of moral worth? They are socially valuable people.

Lottery

A final option identified by Rachel Gillon for choosing between two contenders for the one place on the life-saving machine is that of lottery. You could, she suggested, use 'eenie meenie minee mo'. Assuming that it is fair and unbiased, a lottery offers a way of discriminating between people when choice is no longer morally tolerable. If we are unable to identify any morally relevant differences between the several contenders for a limited availability of care, then chance might be as fair a way as any of discriminating between them. There is more than one way in which a lottery may be carried out. In its 'pure' form, resort could be had to the archetypal toss of a coin, the roll of a dice, or (more realistically) an electronic device for generating random numbers. More weakly, a system of first-come first-served is a lottery of a kind, though it is *not* one in which every contender has an equal chance of selection: those who know about the lottery have an obvious advantage over those who do not, and those for whom the access to care involves a cost are penalized in relation to those facing lower access costs or none at all. But however it may be done, the essence of a lottery is, in Calabresi and Bobbitt's (1978) arresting phrase, that it is 'a choice not to choose' (p. 41).

In favour of a lottery is its obvious aroma of egalitarianism. A lottery, by definition, is blind. Because it has no foreknowledge of those it is selecting (even if they are chosen in the order in which they appear), it cannot *systematically* favour some groups of candidates over others. All are treated alike. It thus removes the possibility of people being chosen on criteria which may not be morally relevant, and it proclaims the incorruptibility of the selection process. Its weakness lies in precisely the obverse side of the coin: a lottery also removes the possibility of people being positively chosen on the basis of criteria which *are* seen as morally relevant. It was this consideration that led Rachel Gillon to reject it as a solution to her problem: 'the one who needed it the most, or the youngest, or the kindest might not get it'. By choosing not to choose, the possibility is created of care going to those who, in moral terms, might not be seen as having a strong claim to priority.

Practical problems would also arise in the application of lottery principles to the rationing of care in complex systems like the NHS. Over what area would the lottery operate? Would there be a single national lottery for, say, all patients needing coronary artery surgery, or would there be separate local lotteries for each health district or even each hospital? A nationwide coverage would uphold the principle of even-handedness throughout the NHS but would, in practice, favour patients who were able and willing to travel for their treatment. A local coverage would avoid this particular problem, but only at the expense of another kind of inequality between patients living in districts or hospital catchment areas with varying capacities for producing the care. And who would be entered into the lottery? Would it be all those with a particular diagnosis, irrespective of severity, or would they be stratified in some way according to the urgency of their condition? If so, why bother with a lottery at all?

In spite of these formidable obstacles of principle and practicality, a serious case in favour of lottery can be – and has been – made in the limited circumstances in which all other acceptable methods of choosing have been exhausted. If it can honestly be said that no further morally relevant criteria remain for choosing between A and B, then the fairest way of proceeding may indeed be by chance. It is, however, difficult to imagine what these circumstances might be. One such set of conditions has been identified by Doyal (1995), whose vision of a morally defensible health care structure is examined in Chapter 3. Doyal would, ideally, have us ration care on the basis of people's needs and nothing else; but he recognizes that a point may eventually be reached at which need ceases to be a practical basis of discrimination. Situations may arise in which no further distinctions can sensibly be made between the needs of patients who are waiting for the same treatment. Where this occurs, Doyal contends, a form of lottery is not merely a last resort that we have to accept *faute de mieux*, it is positively to be desired as a safeguard against the bias or predilections that might otherwise influence the decisions of the doctors who are managing the waiting lists.

Ordering the criteria

In choosing fairly between Dubedat and Blenkinsop (or, more generally, in making the kinds of choices of which Dubedat and Blenkinsop are the representatives), a range of personal qualities might be taken into account. They include need, age, merit, appeal and esteem. They reflect complicated ideas about rights, responsibility, status, altruism, esteem and even-handedness. They are, to a greater or lesser degree, contestable as morally relevant considerations in the fair allocation of health care resources, for as Warnock (1998) has observed, ethics is a matter of judgment and sentiment as well as of reason. They may come into conflict with each other. Where, then, can the arguments go from here?

One or two obvious points can be made. Firstly, some of the criteria that may be brought into the debate may reasonably be dismissed as having little or no moral authority. We may feel able to say with some confidence what is *not* morally acceptable even though we may be less clear about what is. It seems unlikely, for example, that personal appeal or professional prejudice would be widely acceptable as reasons for either choosing or rejecting a prospective patient, any more than gender or ethnicity would be. It surely offends our sense of justice that people's chances of gaining access to the care they need can hinge simply upon whether their faces fit.

Secondly, it seems to be important not only *why* choices are made but also *how* they are made. People's well-being, and in some cases even their lives, may be at stake; and those who control the selection processes have a moral responsibility to act in what they believe to be a responsible and even-handed way. They should not knowingly and deliberately treat a patient unfairly. A moral approach to the processes of choice is the theme of Chapter 4. Beyond that, the question remains: can we say that some criteria, and the principles and values they reflect, have a justifiable priority over others? There are a number of ways of responding to the question.

Moral nihilism

First, we could adopt a position of moral nihilism in one or other of its several forms. Nihilism holds, broadly, that morality is an illusion: nothing is ever right or wrong, just or unjust, good or bad (Harman, 1977). The search for a moral answer to a question is doomed to failure because it does not exist. All that can be done is to examine, debate and test the range of solutions on offer, knowing that each will have its protagonists and antagonists. Some will claim to be pleading from a position of moral authority, others from a stand-point of opportunism or self-interest; but that does not matter, for all who wish to take part are admitted to the cockpit of debate. In the post-modern world they are free to 'tell their stories' and to argue their cases.

From this perspective, the resolutions that emerge reflect nothing more than the degree of power – intellectual, political, professional or otherwise – that those engaged in the debate possess. It cannot reflect the weight of moral opinion because none exists. All that the power structure can do is to adjudicate between competing values and interests; and those with the most clout will carry the day. The outcome will be thought by some to be right and by others wrong; but that is simply the nature of the pluralist world of political power. Those who want their views to prevail would better spend their time lobbying in the corridors of power than studying the texts on ethics.

Moral absolutism

At an opposite extreme, we could assume that some values, far from being contingent, are absolute values that should always take precedence over others – or, at least, that they have immense authority and should be disregarded only in extreme and very carefully considered circumstances. They are to be taken with the utmost seriousness because they have emanated from an immensely authoritative source and they have stood the test of time. Obvious, though not exclusive, exemplars of such values are those contained in religious writings. What Arras (1997) has termed the 'foundational stories' of the monotheistic religions (Islam, Judaism and Christianity) may offer guidelines here, if only negative ones. The Christian New Testament, for example, pays no homage to social standing or financial wealth and it deprecates partiality and prejudice. It cherishes the old and the young alike, and, as the prodigal son found to his advantage, it forgives those who are the architects of their own misfortune. Above all, it enjoins the better off to care for the poor and the dispossessed, not only through the giving of alms but also through the cheerful payment of legally imposed taxes. The ethics of the New Testament, even though yielding up no particular rules for choosing between competing patients, would place a dominant moral emphasis on the care of those at the bottom of the social pile.

To say this, however, is to highlight an obvious difficulty in using absolute values as the basis for moral choices affecting the general public. They are absolute only for those who recognize them as such, and they cannot easily be applied in modern situations of immense complexity that are light-years removed from the cultures in which they originated. Even committed believers might balk at the prospect of a consultant renal physician managing his dialysis facilities with a stethoscope in one hand and the New Testament in the other.

Moral naturalism

A third way forward, lying pragmatically somewhere between the first two, is that of moral naturalism. It accepts neither the nihilist view of an amoral world nor the absolutist belief in given and immutable moral values. Naturalism acknowledges the reality of moral sentiment, but it does so in the context of an intelligent species with an evolutionary history and a complex culture. The influence of Darwinism here is strong. In *The Descent of Man,* Darwin noted that of all the differences between man and the lower animals a sense of morality or conscience was by far the most important (Darwin, 1894). Indeed, Darwin regarded conscience as 'the most noble of all the attributes of man, leading him without a moment's hesitation to risk his life for that of a fellow-creature; or after due deliberation, impelled simply by deep feeling of right or duty, to sacrifice it in some great cause' (*op. cit.*, p. 97). *Homo sapiens* is, by nature, an ethical being. We have an in-built sense that things can be right or wrong, just or unjust.

It is, however, an inescapable consequence of Darwinism that this 'most noble of attributes' has developed through the same evolutionary process of natural selection that has endowed *homo sapiens* with all his other physical, psychological and emotional properties. It could not be otherwise. There is no need to resort either to the religious idea of a God-given system of morality or to a contractarian view of morality in which intelligent men, pursuing their own self-interest, agree to refrain from harming one another (Midgley, 1994). This, Darwin argued, could not possibly be right, for long before humanity ever existed there were social animals which had begun to love and help those around them, not for reasons of prudence but out of simple natural affection. Such affection, allied to an expanding cerebral cortex that allowed *homo sapiens* to reflect upon the effects of his behaviour on others and to develop feelings of remorse and regret, is explanation enough.

The way of moral naturalism implies the existence in some sense of reservoirs of shared moral sensitivity among human beings, just as there are reservoirs of shared genes, instincts, and (as Jung would have it) memories. The sense of justice is not merely an abstract construct: it is a real experience. We really do have some feeling of what is right or wrong, just or unjust, acceptable or unacceptable. We really can distinguish between what we *ought* to do and what we *want* to do, even when the two come into conflict; and it may be this 'natural' sense of justice that leads us to reject partiality and prejudice as a proper basis for choosing between individuals. There is a feeling 'in our bones' that it would be wrong to reject a patient for treatment *simply* because her face didn't fit with the clinical team. It seems 'obviously' right to us that more medical time should be devoted to the young woman with breast cancer than the lonely old man with a sore throat. We 'naturally' accept that honesty is right and mendacity is wrong, even though we may encounter particular circumstances in which it appears to be, and may actually be, in our interests to lie. These might be seen as default values: they define the way in which we think things *ought* to be done. They are not values that we have, either literally or metaphorically, contracted to uphold; they are part of the very fabric of humanity.

A way forward?

Can anything of value be said about these three perspectives that might begin to shed some light upon the problem of primacy among the competing criteria with which this chapter has been concerned? Should we attempt to choose between individuals in the light of what we believe to be the authoritative values of a 'foundational story'? Should we choose in the light of the arguments that can best withstand the tempering heat of critical debate? Or should we choose in the light of strong cultural values that have stood the test of time and that seem broadly to correspond with well founded and widely shared views of what is fair and just?

It is tempting to argue that reason can take us no farther, for this is a question to which there is no answer. It reduces to a matter of values which, ultimately, can be neither attacked nor defended. Yet there may be a little more to be said than that. Moral nihilism, absolutism and naturalism do not, in practice, seem to have an equal status or authority in public discourse. Nor do they seem to strike informed observers as equally attractive. Nihilism is a rather gloomy way of looking at ourselves, and it does not accord well with our ordinary ways of talking and thinking. Most people, when observed in their daily lives, do appear to have a sense that something may be right or wrong as well as, say, stupid or shrewd. Absolutism, by contrast, may offer a more hopeful perspective on life, but its precepts are by definition non-negotiable. We have to take them or leave them. They demand an unconditional acceptance, with little allowance for circumstance. Naturalism, the 'third way', is plainly attractive precisely because it avoids such problems. It is also seemingly widely accepted. Singer (1994) regards Darwin's account of the origins of morality as 'the general outline of what is surely the right answer to the question' (p. 20). Yet it needs to be handled with care, having the apparent capacity to collapse into either nihilism or absolutism if we try to make it do too much. It is precisely to avoid this trap that we shall have to revisit the issue in the context of the 'stories' told in Chapter 6.

Note

Extracts from *The Doctor's Dilemma*, by G.B. Shaw (1939) are reprinted by permission of The Society of Authors, on behalf of the Bernard Shaw Estate.

3

Ethics and the structures of health care rationing

Structure, process and outcome

The previous chapter considered an important strand in the literature on the moral bases of rationing in health care, namely the grounds for distinguishing between individual patients when resources are insufficient to treat them all. There are, however, other writings that offer us a different moral perspective on the problem, and it to these that the next three chapters turn. They are arranged loosely around the distinction drawn by Donabedian (1980) between the structures, the processes and the outcomes of health care. The distinction is reasonably straightforward, though the categories are by no means watertight and the allocation of ideas to one or the other is to some extent arbitrary.

The *structures* of health care comprise the various components of the organizational framework through which health care is delivered. The basic characteristics of health care structures are, in Donabedian's view, that they are relatively stable and that they influence the kind of care that is provided (*op. cit.*, p. 81). The moral question that is usually asked about the structures of care in the context of rationing is whether they are fair. Given that health services will always be in short supply in relation to the potential demand for them, are they structured and organized in ways that will promote rather than diminish people's fair and equitable access to them? What does equitable mean in this context? And what might such a structural framework look like?

The *processes* of health care describe the ways in which the provision of care is actually carried out. They may cover a wide swathe of activity, from the ways in which governments and health authorities set about managing the gap between supply and demand to the ways in which clinicians deal with their patients. The moral question that is usually asked about the processes of care is whether they are ethical. Given that governments and health authorities can never provide enough resources to meet everyone's needs for care, are the bases of their decisions ethically defensible? Given that doctors, nurses and other practitioners are unable to do all that they may wish to do for their patients, are they making clinical choices in ways that correspond with established ethical criteria?

The *outcomes* of care are, self-evidently, the results or the effects of care. Outcomes may be thought of in terms either of individual patients or of groups of patients, and they may conflict. If a choice can be made between a large benefit for a small number of patients (for example by prescribing a life-saving but expensive drug) or a smaller benefit for a larger number of patients (for example by low-cost services that improve the length or quality of many people's lives), are there any morally acceptable criteria that might aid the choice? Are some outcomes morally to be preferred to others?

This chapter addresses the question of equity in the structures of health care. Can we identify the features of a health care system that are acceptable as evidence of its fairness? What does 'fair' mean in this context? And what might such a system look like? The questions are examined through the work of four writers whose arguments are particularly pertinent to the ways in which health care services are structured: John Rawls, Norman Daniels, Len Doyal and Robert Nozick. The first three have been chosen because their work builds upon each other's: Daniels tries to develop Rawls' high-level theory in the particular context of health care, and Doyal's work can be read as an attempt to imagine how Daniels' insights might find their expression through the organizational framework of the NHS. Nozick's earlier writing has been selected to illustrate the libertarian counter-arguments about the almost taken-for-granted assumptions in the others' works about the legitimate use of state power to enforce and sustain particular structures of care.

Rawls' theory of justice

Justice and primary goods

Rawls' *A Theory of Justice*, published in 1971, has achieved an enormous impact not only in academic cloisters but in many areas of public and human service where questions of fairness arise. As Nozick later observed in a context that was critical of certain aspects of Rawls' ideas, 'political philosophers now must either work with Rawls' theory or explain why not' (Nozick, 1974, p. 183). Rawls' book is voluminous in size and vast in the range and scale of its argument, and although only the briefest of summaries can be given here, the core of his analysis can fairly well be understood in abbreviated form.

Rawls begins by noting that many different kinds of things are said to be just or unjust, including big things such as laws, institutions and social systems and little things such as people's attitudes, judgments and actions (Rawls, 1971, p. 7). His particular concern, however, is with what he calls 'social justice' – that is, the way in which society is *structured*, including its major social, political, legal and economic institutions. Compendious though this focus is, it is important because it is through these institutions that people's chances in life are influenced. People do not begin the competition of life from the same starting-point: because of the ways in which the major social institutions work, some people are much more handicapped than others. Yet such inequalities, Rawls argues, cannot possibly be justified by appealing to the notions of merit or desert. Unmerited inequality is built into the basic structures of human society, hampering some people and advantaging others at birth and throughout life. Injustice is, at root, a structural problem; and Rawls sets himself the task of finding a robust set of criteria that must be satisfied before any social structure can be considered just.

Rawls' theory is concerned, at heart, with the ways in which a just social structure would allocate a set of what he calls 'primary social goods'. Such goods would include rights and liberties, powers and opportunities, income and wealth (*op. cit.*, p. 62). They are primary goods because they are things that every rational person is presumed to want, whatever they may hope or plan to get out of life. Rawls acknowledges the presence of other kinds of primary goods, including 'natural goods' such as health and vigour, intelligence and imagination; but the distribution of these, he argues, is less determined by the basic social structure. A just society, then, would be one in which its basic social structures were so arranged that everyone had a fair share of the 'primary social goods'.

Rawls' principles

The principle of greatest equal liberty

So far so good; but how would a just society, as Rawls defines it, be recognized? Rawls proposes two (in fact three) principles that, if fully met, would qualify a society as being just. The first is what he calls the *principle of greatest equal liberty*. In its final formulation, this principle states that 'each person is to have an equal right to the most extensive total system of equal basic liberties compatible with a similar system of liberty for all' (*op. cit.*, p. 302). Everyone should have an equal right to as extensive a menu of basic liberties as possible, including, for example, the freedom of speech and assembly, the right to vote and hold public office, and the freedom from arbitrary arrest. (The right to good health, or even to good health care, is not among the menu of liberties.) But the extent of the menu of basic liberties must be subordinate to the principle that everyone must have an equal right to the same menu. Liberties cannot be extended for some if the cost of doing so is their exclusion for others.

The difference principle

Rawls' second principle is sub-divided into two – hence the convention of regarding his theory as comprising three principles in all. The first part, which Rawls calls the *difference principle*, states that 'social and economic inequalities are to be arranged so that they are . . . to the greatest benefit of the least advantaged . . .' (*op. cit.*, p. 302). Whereas the principle of greatest equal liberty is concerned with the distribution of basic liberties, the difference principle is concerned with the distribution of another sub-set of primary goods – social goods (power and authority) and economic goods (wealth and income). The least advantaged people referred to in the difference principle are those with the lowest prospects of enjoying such goods.

Importantly, the principle allows the possibility that an unequal share-out of social and economic goods may be compatible with a just distribution – but only if it works to the advantage of the least advantaged members of the society. The touchstone of the difference principle is the *absolute* opportunity that is available to the least advantaged to enjoy power, authority, income and wealth. Further inequalities in the way such goods are distributed can be justified under the difference principle – but only if they improve the real lot of those at the bottom of the pile.

A serious difficulty with the difference principle, which Rawls explicitly acknowledges, is that of defining the least advantaged people in any relevant population (*op. cit.*, p. 98). Here, he avers, it is impossible to avoid a certain degree of arbitrariness; and he offers two solutions. One solution involves the notion of the 'representative worst-off man', who can be identified by taking a particular social group, such as unskilled workers, and then regarding the representative as the average of that group. The other solution is to regard all those with incomes below the average of the whole group as being the least advantaged. The difficulty of identifying the least advantaged people in any group is not a minor one for Rawls. His agenda is not only theoretical; it is also concerned with advancing the cause of justice in real-life contexts, and this can be done only if the principles that define a just distribution of primary social goods can be put to practical use. It requires not only a theoretically robust definition of justice but also one that can be applied to real people in real situations in real societies.

The principle of fair equality of opportunity

The second part of Rawls' second principle, which he calls the *principle of fair equality of opportunity*, states that 'social and economic inequalities are to be arranged so that they are attached to offices and positions open to all under conditions of fair equality of opportunity' (*op. cit.*, p. 302). To the extent that inequalities exist in the distribution of social and economic goods throughout a society, they should be capable of being overcome through institutions to which everyone has an equal and fair chance of access. The labour market is an obvious exemplar of such an institution, since it is through the world of paid employment that most people earn their incomes and are able to accumulate their wealth. The principle of fair equality of opportunity would require people to have an equal chance of getting jobs relative to their capacity to do them. It would not, for instance, require someone with no formal educational qualifications to have the same chance of being appointed a professor as someone with higher academic qualifications; but it would require that an applicant with the relevant qualifications should not be overlooked because of gender, sexual orientation, religion or other characteristics that are intrinsically unrelated to the capacity to do the job.

Justifying the principles

Rawls' three principles and two rules about the defining features of a just social structure are stated as ethical imperatives: that is, they assert that a society which systematically sought to embody them *would* be a just society, and, by implication, that each society *should* be structured in this way. But why? Why are these particular principles and rules, and not others, postulated as the defining hallmarks of justice? Why, especially, is Rawls' system claimed to be superior to utilitarian approaches (see

Chapter 5) which proclaim that justice lies in securing the greatest benefit of the greatest number of people?

Rawls answers such questions in two ways – through an appeal to people's considered moral judgments about what is just or unjust, or, if this fails, through what he describes as 'persuasion by philosophical reflection' (*op. cit.*, p. 21). In this he appeals to Kant's notion of the autonomous agent, motivated by rational principles rather than personal or particular desires. It is the first of these approaches to the question of validity that has attracted the greater interest.

Matching judgments

Rawls argues that his principles and rules can be held to be valid if they match up to the considered moral judgments that people *actually* make about what is just or unjust in society. They are also valid if they match up to the considered judgments that people *would* make *if* they were made under circumstances which are appropriate for deciding what is just and what is unjust. The requirement that such judgments must be 'considered' judgments is an important one: implicit in the whole of Rawls' approach is the assumption that the business of making moral choices is a serious matter and that only the views of those who engage in it in a serious and studied way can be taken into account. The bar-room philosopher, tanked up and playing to a goading audience, is not a relevant source of wisdom or insight.

So Rawls' first justification for his principles and rules is simply that they correspond to people's *actual* reflective views about what is just and unjust in society. Ultimately, his system rests on an appeal to the moral sentiments of the people. A general example of this would flow from his concern, in the difference principle, not only to maximize the overall amount of wealth and income in society but also to protect the position of those at the bottom of the social pile. Widening inequalities in income and wealth might well be achievable at the expense of a worsening in the position of those who are very poor; but this would be identified as an unjust act by the difference principle. In contrast, classical utilitarianism has no such concern with the least advantaged: its only mission is to maximize the *total* amount of benefit in a society, whatever the cost to those with the least enjoyment of it (see Chapter 5). It is the former approach, Rawls would have to argue, that better corresponds with people's considered views about what is just. On mature reflection, people would not consider a structure which ignored the plight of the least advantaged to be a just one.

Matching circumstances

But Rawls has a fall-back position in case this argument is rejected. The validity of his principles and rules, he argues, can also be established by their correspondence not only with the considered moral judgments that people *actually* make, but also with those that they *would* make under suitable circumstances. He describes his principles as those that 'free and rational persons, concerned to further their own interests, would accept in an initial position of equality as defining the fundamental terms of their association' (*op. cit.*, p. 11). Rawls is here drawing upon the time-hallowed idea of a social contract, either real or metaphorical, into which people voluntarily enter to regulate the major relationships between them; but he takes the idea into new territory by trying to imagine a society in which everyone is equally in the dark and then asking what, in such an imaginary society, people would contractually accept as a fair way of organizing themselves.

The original position

Assumptions of the original position

One of the most widely publicized elements in Rawls' system has been his conception of the imaginary society – the 'original position', as he terms it – from which he believes his principles of justice would naturally spring. It contains four assumptions. First, those who are party to the contract are assumed to be rational people pursuing their life plans in a rational way. In particular, Rawls assumes that they will want to own the largest possible share of the primary goods (wealth, power, income, etc.) because these are basic prerequisites for achieving any goals or ambitions. Second, the inhabitants of this imagined society are deprived of information about their own position within it. They do not know if they are rich or poor, black or white, weak or strong, male or female. Therefore, as rational people, they will not try to engineer a set of social relationships which systematically benefit some at the expense of others, for they do not know whether they themselves will be within the favoured groups. White people would not be favoured over black people, or men over women, because the parties to the contract might eventually find themselves to be black or female. Rawls calls this the 'veil of ignorance' (*op. cit.*, p. 136).

The other two assumptions inherent in the 'original position' are less dramatic. The principles of justice that are chosen by the parties to the social contract must have certain features that enable them to work effectively as principles. They must, for example, be generalized principles that are universally applied, perfectly publicized and capable of acting as a final court of appeal for settling disputes about the justice of any particular act. And finally, the people must have a free choice of the principles that will form the basis of the society in which they are to live, including other, rival principles (such as classical utilitarianism). With all these conditions met, Rawls argues, people will indeed choose his principles of social justice in preference to any others that are on offer. But why?

The maximin rule

The main answer, Rawls proposes, lies in what he calls the 'maximin rule', which states that, when faced with choices from within the veil of ignorance, rational people who are bent on advancing their own interests will choose the option in which the most disastrous result is the least damaging for them. As Rawls puts it, 'the maximin rule tells us to rank alternatives by their worst possible outcomes: we are to adopt the alternative in which the worst possible outcome is superior to the worst outcomes of the others' (*op. cit.*, pp. 152–3). Thus, people in the 'original position' will choose his principles in preference to utilitarianism because they will know that the worst that could happen to them under a Rawlsian contract would be better than the worst that could happen under a utilitarian contract.

Utilitarianism, for example, allows the liberties of some to be severely restricted if the result is a greater overall liberty for many. People within the veil of ignorance, not knowing about their positions in society, might, if they chose a utilitarian contract, find themselves disenfranchised, in slavery, denied the freedom of speech, subject to arbitrary arrest, or even worse. The least advantaged under utilitarianism may be very badly off indeed. That is why, Rawls argues, the rational person would choose his principles in preference to any others, for the principle of greatest equal liberty requires people to have an *equal* right to as extensive a menu of basic liberties as possible.

Illustrative applications

General practice fund-holding

Although most of Rawls' book is occupied with the abstract theory of his system of justice, some space is given (particularly in Chapter 5) to a consideration of its applications in real-life social institutions. It is this part of his work that has attracted much critical attention, not least because of the intrinsic difficulties involved in applying a huge macrotheory of justice to the detailed structures of local services and institutions. In particular for our purposes, there is no specific reference in Rawls' work to social justice in relation to the distribution and accessibility of health care.

Yet Rawls' theory of justice is sufficiently precise to allow a measure of application of his principles to issues of a moral nature in health care, and to enable specific conclusions to be drawn from them. An example might be the debate within the NHS in the early 1990s about the fairness of fund-holding (FH) in general practice. For several years following the introduction of the scheme in 1991, concerns were expressed about the steady development of a dual standard of service – one for patients registered with FH practices and a lower one for other patients (White-head, 1994, p. 215). Anecdotal stories accumulated (Coulter, 1995), later supported by a measure of empirical evidence (Dowling, 1997), that the former were receiving faster, and possibly better, care from hospitals when they were referred to them. Such findings, and the conclusions that may validly be drawn from them, must be treated with caution (Powell, 1997, p. 147); but to the extent that they validly reveal the shifts induced by the FH experiment, they are evidence of widening inequalities in people's access to good hospital care. Any such inequalities, moreover, are largely unmerited, since people in many parts of the country have a limited choice about the GP with whom they are registered. If people live outside the catchment zone of any FH practice, or if all the local FH practices have closed their books to new registrations, the resultant inequalities must simply be borne with placid acceptance.

Rawls' theory of justice, however, does not unconditionally condemn existing or even widening inequalities of access. Quite the reverse: under the difference principle they would be justified if they worked to the benefit of the least advantaged – provided that the other principles, particularly the principle of greatest equal liberty, were not violated in the process. And in the case of fund-holding, this appears to be precisely what has occurred: FH practices have indeed succeeded in sharpening up the service given by the provider hospitals, but, together with other government policies such as the Patient's Charter and the waiting list initiatives, they have also enhanced the service received by patients in non-FH practices (Audit Commission, 1996). Inequalities in access to hospital care may have increased, but those with the poorest access have often received a better deal in absolute terms. Any increase in inequality is therefore justifiable under the difference principle because it has improved the lot of the least advantaged without harming their liberties.

Utilitarianism and the case of Jaymee Bowen

In a more diffuse way, Rawls' analysis draws our attention to a number of features of health care structures that might, in the light of his ideas, raise moral questions about their justice. His entire approach is deeply and deliberately antithetical to the classical utilitarian view that the aims of justice are served by securing the greatest happiness of the greatest number, however much unhappiness there may be among those who are passed over in the process. It was just such a utilitarian perspective that lay at the heart of the Court of Appeal's decision in the case of Jaymee Bowen (see Chapters 1 and 4) that a health authority would be justified in refusing to fund a particular treatment if it believed that a greater good would result from using the funds elsewhere (Price, 1996). The Court held, in floridly utilitarian language, that 'difficult and agonising judgements have to be made as to how a limited budget is best allocated to the maximum advantage of the maximum number of patients' (*op. cit.*, p. 167).

Rawls' theory, by contrast, asserts that a utilitarian approach cannot, of itself, assure a just distribution of primary social goods. The difference principle requires the interests of the least advantaged never to be sacrificed for a greater collective good. Of course, since Rawls excludes health care from his catalogue of primary social goods, there can be no simple or straightforward application of his ideas to the problem in hand. Nevertheless, the principles upon which his theory is constructed find sympathetic echoes in other contemporary debates about the allocation of health care and they may profit from a careful application in this field. One who has attempted the task is Daniels.

Daniels' theory of the fair equality of opportunity

Health care and distributional justice

Daniels, a neo-Rawlsian American philosopher, has tried over many years to construct an approach to the fair allocation of health care that takes account of wider established theories about distributional justice (Daniels, 1985, 1988; Daniels, Light and Caplan, 1996). Daniels begins by posing the question of why a concern with distributional justice should extend to health care at all. What is it about health care that makes it morally more important than many other things which improve the quality of people's lives? His initial answer lies in an appeal to public sentiment: people seem to feel that health care is sufficiently important to personal well-being that its availability should be determined by nothing other than medical need. Non-medical features, particularly those to do with social or economic fortune, should not determine people's access to care.

But this raises the question: access to what? Should medical need determine people's access to the *entire* spectrum of services offered by a modern health care system, or only to some segments of it – those, perhaps, which represent a basic minimum core of services? If justice requires access to health care to be based on medical need alone, the question arises of *which* needs should be met when it is not possible to meet them all? The answer, Daniels proposes, must lie in a sharper, more discriminating definition of the concept of need. Justice can hardly require the satisfaction of each and every need for health care, however trivial it may be. After all, Rawls did not require his theory of justice to encompass all kinds of social goods, merely those that were of primary significance in the lives of ordinary people. The object of justice, Daniels maintains, is not to ensure universal happiness or satisfaction but to provide a fair and acceptable framework within which people can be enabled to pursue their own expectations of happiness, whether these are extravagant or frugal (Daniels, 1985, p. 38).

It is the idea of 'enablement' that seems to have given Daniels the key to the question, for at the heart of his scheme of distributional justice is the hypothesis that needs are special, giving rise to a moral claim on the resources of the health care system, when – but only when – they are necessary to sustain what he calls 'species-typical normal functioning' (*op. cit.*, p. 26). Some health care needs – but only some – are special because, unless they are met, they threaten the opportunities that people have for constructing their 'life plans'.

The actual content of people's life plans – what they hope or expect to do with their lives – is of no material consequence. For all manner of reasons that social policy cannot and should not seek to influence, people vary enormously in what they wish to achieve in their lives. It matters not that some have lofty aspirations to wealth, power or fame and others have more modest goals around their work, homes, families and pensions. People also vary in the talents, interests, aptitudes and abilities that bear upon their choices in life. These can be set aside, for there is little that public policy can do to alter them. What *does* matter is that, simply by virtue of being human, people should have a fair and equal opportunity to try to achieve *whatever it is they want to achieve*. And to the extent that illness or disability detracts from such opportunity, people's needs become ones that have a moral claim for resolution. As Daniels puts it, 'impairment of normal functioning through disease and disability restricts an individual's opportunity *relative to that portion of the normal range his skills and talents would have made available to him were he healthy'* (*op. cit.*, pp. 33–4, italics in original). A life plan is simply that through which, apart from illness or disability, each person can reasonably expect to find satisfaction, fulfilment and happiness. 'My conclusion', Daniels argues, 'is that we should use impairment of the normal opportunity range as a fairly crude measure of the relative importance of health care needs . . . It will be more important to prevent, cure or compensate for those diseases which involve a greater curtailment of an individual's share of the normal opportunity range' (1985, p. 35).

Daniels and Rawls

There are, as Daniels himself recognizes, close similarities between his approach to social justice and that of Rawls. Both are contractarians and both are engaged in a quest for higher-order principles of justice that can be applied in the different contexts in which questions about a fair allocation of scarce resources arise. For Rawls, the crux of the principle lies in the welfare of those who are least advantaged; for Daniels it lies in the opportunities that people have for achieving their ambitions in life. If Rawls can be said to be an egalitarian, Daniels is an opportunity-maximizer. Yet Daniels explicitly acknowledges his debt to Rawls, even to the extent of trying to apply Rawls' theory more directly than he does himself to the arena of health care.

Having noted that Rawls excludes health from his compendium of social goods, Daniels proposes that Rawls' ideas can be extended to health care by the simple expedient of including health care organizations among the basic arrangements in society that help to promote a fair equality of opportunity. 'Health care institutions', he suggests, 'help to provide the framework of liberties and opportunities within which individuals can use their fair income shares to pursue their own conception of the good' (*op. cit.*, p. 47). By subsuming the health care system within Rawls' principle of fair equality of opportunity in this way, Daniels is adhering as closely as he can to the conditions of Rawls' imaginary original position, in which people are normal, fully functioning individuals with a complete life span.

Objections

Having set out his theory of fair equality of opportunity, Daniels then defends it from objections that may be raised against it. Firstly, he deals with the charge that health and medical care services meet many other kinds of human needs in addition to those that adversely affect people's opportunities in life. The reduction of pain, suffering and misery would be one such aim of medical care, even though pain and suffering may not always prevent people from achieving their life plans. Daniels concedes that this is of course true; but he argues that, by focusing on needs which *do* detract from people's opportunities, his theory is capable of discriminating between services and treatments that can and cannot properly be the subject of moral concern.

> My account abstracts from these varied effects of health care a central function – the maintenance of species-typical functional organisation – and emphasises its central effect on opportunity. My contention is that most uses of health care services which we intuitively find important, such as those in which we seek to reduce pain, will be encompassed by this central effect on opportunity. (*op. cit.*, pp. 49–50)

Secondly, Daniels confronts the charge that his theory of fair equality of opportunity is either too vague or too broad. It is one thing to theorize about the relationship between people's health and their opportunities to pursue their life plans; it is rather more difficult to identify the *particular* ways in which the relationship works. In any case it is now conceded, even by governments, that other goods and services, including income, education and mobility, probably have a greater impact on people's opportunities to pursue their life plans than health and medical care (Department of Health, 1998). Daniels concedes the truth of this and accepts that it puts him in a more difficult position than Rawls, who limits his own notion of equal opportunity to people's access to those institutions, such as the labour market, which affect their capacity to enjoy the primary social and economic goods. His rather timid defence is that certain institutions, including health care, *do* meet needs which 'quite generally have a central impact on individual shares of the normal opportunity range and which should therefore be governed directly by the opportunity principle' (*op. cit.*, p. 52).

Thirdly, and contrariwise, the charge may be made that Daniels' account is too strong. It may be objected, he says, that he is trying to eliminate individual differences between people by reducing them to a uniform level of achievement in the struggles of life. To this he pleads not guilty: a fair equality of opportunity is not one in which all are restricted to the same segments of the spectrum of opportunity. Rather, opportunity is equal when everyone is equally spared the kinds of impediments (including ill health and disability) that hinder their attainment of whatever their own personal goals may be (*op. cit.*, p. 52). Nor, Daniels claims, does his account require so much money to be spent on the bottomless pit of health care need that other worthy social goals might suffer from fiscal neglect. In his scheme of things, old people would have no right to expect, say, cryogenic preservation because that would lie far outside the range of normal species functioning. Daniels is careful to stress that he is not arguing for any particular quantum of health care as a right, merely that, within the resources available to them, health care institutions should allocate those resources in accordance with his general principles governing people's equality of opportunity.

Age and the theory of fair equality of opportunity

Some of the most interesting passages in Daniels' writing are those in which he applies his theory to current problems in the allocation of health care resources. The broad conclusion to be drawn from his exposition is that health care institutions should be structured in ways that offer equal protection for all against the threats that illness and disability pose to people's opportunity of enjoying 'normal species functioning'. But what might this mean in particular contexts? One such context, which Daniels explores in much detail, is that of age (Daniels, 1988).

The role of age in the just structure of services

Questions about the relevance of age as a morally defensible criterion for the allocation of health care resources run like a repetitive motif through many of the debates about distributional justice (see Chapter 2). Is it fair, in sharing out the resources that are available for health care, to discriminate against older people simply because of their age? Conventional answers are polarized. One response is positive: yes, it is fair (Williams, 1997). Priority should be given to the young in the rationing of life-extending services because the old have already had their chance of living a goodly number of years and fairness requires a similar chance to be given to their successors. The other response is negative: no, it is not fair (Grimley Evans, 1997). Justice requires people to be treated according to their needs, and other criteria such as age, gender and ethnicity are morally irrelevant to the decision about who to treat.

Daniels' theory of fair equality of opportunity leads him to an interestingly different perspective on the problem. He first notes that age is not, in fact, the same as gender or ethnicity: unlike these two personal properties, which remain constant throughout life, age changes (Daniels, 1988, p. 40). People get older the longer they live. An obvious but frequently overlooked conclusion to be drawn from this commonplace observation is that, if the young are always treated generously and the old are always treated parsimoniously, then over a normal life span each individual receives both generous *and* parsimonious treatment. The question does not arise of whether it is fair to give generous treatment to one category of people and parsimonious treatment to another category: both kinds of treatments are given to the *same* people, but at different stages in their lives. Morally, therefore, it is false to counterpoise the treatment of young people against that of old people. If everyone is treated fairly at each stage of their lives, then over a full lifetime all will receive fair treatment.

The 'prudential life-span account'

It is this trite but intriguing observation about the progression of people's ages that leads Daniels to what he calls the 'prudential life-span account'. At the core of the account is the interesting proposition that the allocation of health care resources is not only a cross-sectional problem but also a longitudinal one. It is not merely a matter of who gets what at any particular moment in time, but more importantly of who gets what across a normal span of life. Health care systems, Daniels suggests, can be structured in such a way that they allocate care differentially over a lifetime, and the more that is allocated in the earlier years, the less will be available for allocation in later years.

Health policy may, for example, invest heavily in services for children and young people, resulting in low infant mortality rates and a high proportion of people living through to old age. Under such a policy, people will draw more heavily on their fair share of care earlier in life and less in later life. The cost, however, will be a lighter investment in services for older people, probably resulting in a lowered proportion of old people who reach a very advanced age. Alternatively, health policy may redistribute care more aggressively across the normal life-span, allocating rather less in the earlier years and more in the later years. There is, in short, an opportunity for trade-off between, on the one hand, the prospect of large numbers of people reaching old age but few reaching very old age, and, on the other, the prospect of fewer people reaching old age but proportionally more of these attaining a very advanced age.

Life stages and the theory of fair equality of opportunity

The question then arises of how the justice of these alternatives, and an infinite variety of intermediate positions, is to be determined. In answering it, Daniels draws directly from his theory of 'fair equality of opportunity'. The key realization, he argues, is that the notion of fair equality of opportunity can be applied not in a uniform way across an entire lifetime but in different ways at different stages in life (*op. cit.*, pp. 73–4). For most people, he suggests, life is divided into a number of fairly homogenous stages: nurturing and training in childhood and youth; building careers and raising families in the middle years of adulthood; easing up and winding down in the later years. The normal range of opportunities that are open to people is different at each stage, and so too is the function of the health care system in maximizing people's opportunities.

The possibility arises, of course, that people will vary in the opportunity investments they would wish to make at different stages in their lives. Some will prefer to invest most heavily in the early years of childhood and youth, believing that it is in these years that their basic life-chances are determined; others may give a higher priority to the middle years of life, reasoning that it is at this stage that the greatest opportunities and rewards are likely to be available – provided they have the health to enjoy them; and some may opt for old age, since this is the time of life when they are most likely to suffer ill heath and disability and most likely also to be dependent on the services that others provide for them. Is there any moral basis for judging between these alternatives?

Prudent deliberators

In considering this question, Daniels draws heavily upon Rawls' earlier work on the 'original position'. He invites us to imagine a group of 'prudent deliberators' whose task it is to devise a health care structure based upon the principle of the lifetime allocation of resources. Like Rawls' occupants of the original position, Daniels' prudent deliberators are hedged around with constraints (*op. cit.*, pp. 74–5). Firstly, they must find a principled way of designing health care institutions that can distribute resources fairly over each person's life-span. Secondly, they must concern themselves only with services that are instrumental in securing people's fair equality of opportunity. Thirdly, the distributions with which they are to concern themselves must be made across the stages of life, not between persons. Fourthly (following Rawls' striking notion of the 'veil of ignorance') they must not know either the current stage that their lives have reached or the number of stages that remain to them. And finally, they must have a prudent regard for all the stages of life, not a reckless predilection for any one stage.

The prudent deliberators must also have knowledge – far more, it appears, than Rawls would allow the inhabitants of his 'original position'. The deliberators must understand the demographic and epide-miological profiles of their society; they must be familiar with the links between services and opportunities; they must have at least a passing acquaintance with patterns of family support for elderly parents, female participation in the labour force and the stability and mobility of families; and they must be capable of forming a life plan for themselves, either a general plan for the whole of life or (preferably) a differentiated plan for different stages.

Under these constraints, Daniels argues, prudent deliberators would choose a health care structure that gave them the greatest opportunities at the stages in their lives that *they themselves* judged to be of the greatest importance to them (*op. cit.*, p. 94). They would have no need to engage in the interminable debate about the relative fairness of investing more in young people than old people or vice versa, for they would themselves be both young and old. Their only concern would be to allocate their lifetime share of resources, stage by stage, in ways that reflected *their own* priorities about the opportunities they wished to have at each stage. The structure they chose, therefore, would be a morally just one, for it would give priority at *each* stage in the life-cycle to services that fairly protected the normal range of opportunities open to people in their society *at that stage*; and it would do so in proportion to the importance that people attached to different stages. As Daniels puts it, health care would be distributed 'in a way that protects individuals' fair share of the age-relative normal opportunity range for their society. This is the overarching principle that constrains all further deliberation about prudent life-span allocation of health care' (*op. cit.*, p. 76).

'Is age a morally relevant category?' revisited

There is, of course, a large and difficult gulf between the abstract principle and its application in real situations of choice; and it is a gulf that Daniels scarcely attempts to bridge. The principle does, however, lead him to an interesting position on the abiding question of whether age is or is not a morally relevant characteristic in thinking about the fair distribution of resources. Daniels adopts neither of the conventional polarities in the literature. Far from being a morally irrelevant category, he argues, age would be of primary moral importance if the prudent deliberators chose an investment strategy that was markedly biased towards *either* the earlier stages *or* the later stages of life (*op. cit.*, p. 98). If, in other words, people freely chose to phase their access to health care in such a way that their maximum entitlement to it occurred either when they were young or when they were old, then age would rightly become a major criterion for allocating care – provided, of course, that people had the same aggregate opportunities in life whatever the stages at which they chose to take them.

But if they assigned no such bias to the differing stages of life, age would cease to be a morally relevant category. This perspective, as Daniels himself observes, differs markedly from the uncomplicated egalitarian view that people should never be discriminated against for reasons only of age (*op. cit.*, p. 99). Indeed, it is possible, Daniels suggests, to imagine a set of circumstances under which it would be unfair *not* to discriminate on the grounds of age. If, under some imaginary contract, people chose voluntarily to make the greatest use of the health care system in their younger years, and if they all experienced an equal opportunity to fulfil their life plans at those ages, then fairness would actually *require* them to be discriminated against in their later years in favour of the next generation of young citizens. (In passing, Daniels briefly explores the extension of this idea to other areas also in which 'ageism' is conventionally deplored, including access to the labour market.)

Applications

As with Rawls' theory, it is far from easy to take Daniels' ideas away from the drawing board of principle and apply them on the building site of real life. Arresting though his 'prudential life-span account' might be, its application is difficult to envisage in real contexts in which investment choices have to be made in health care. As he rightly concedes, people acting as prudent deliberators may properly disagree about the weights they want to attach to different stages in life: some may be eager children at heart, wanting their cake when they are young; others may be fearful geriatrics, preferring to wait until an age when no other crumbs of comfort are available. The health care system, however, cannot discriminate on such a personal basis. It has to provide a range of services for everyone, and if it exhibits too great a bias towards the needs of one particular age group, it lays itself open to the charge of discrimination against those with differing preferences.

Perhaps the most radically interesting application of Daniels' ideas (though it is not one that he himself pursues) is the notion of a 'lifetime ration book', which would give everyone the guarantee of a fair quantum of care throughout their lives (based on the principle of fair equality of opportunity) but would leave it to each person's individual choice as to when the coupons or vouchers were redeemed. The nearest that British social policy has come to such a project has been its flirtation with vouchers and with the notion of personal or stakeholder capital in pensions and in social security rights. Insurance-based health care systems also reflect the cognate idea of personal entitlement to benefit, as and when the insured person chooses, in relation to the premium credits that have been accumulated. The administrative and moral implications of the lifetime ration book are shuddering even to contemplate, but the idea certainly appears to be faithful to Daniels' view of a just structure of health care.

Doyal's theory of human need

Health care as a proper focus of moral concern

The challenge of trying to give a measure of form and substance to Daniels' ideas has been taken up by Doyal, a British ethicist whose work comes close to providing a concrete illustration of what a morally defensible health care structure might look like (Doyal, 1995). One of Doyal's central aims is a rebuttal of the conclusion reached by the House of Commons Health Committee in 1995 that 'there is no such thing as . . . a correct way of setting priorities' (House of Commons Health Committee, 1995, p. 57). Quite the reverse: Doyal argues that, if priorities are to be set fairly and rationing is to be carried out along equitable lines, then we can identify certain methods of rationing that are manifestly unfair and sketch out others that satisfy a reasonable notion of equity. Among the former are those that rely on measures of cost-benefit ratios (see Chapter 5) and on publicly articulated preferences (see Chapter 4). Techniques which claim to provide a morally acceptable basis for choice by identifying the ratio of benefits to costs for different procedures in fact offend our sense of justice, Doyal claims, for they always accord a low priority to people whose expectations of health following treatment are poor: the very old, the chronically sick, and the long-term handicapped. Likewise, those that consciously reflect the moral values of the local community fall foul of the plurality of public opinion and the sharp social bias inherent in all known methods of tapping it (Doyal, 1993).

Doyal's approach is different. His starting point is similar to Daniels': health care is a proper focus of moral concern because good physical and mental health are necessary conditions for people to participate fully in their society. In place of Daniels' clumsy phrase 'species-typical normal functioning', Doyal speaks of 'flourishing'. People flourish best as human beings when they are able to play a full part in social life, and for this they need to be as healthy as possible. It is not simply a selfish matter of needing care for one's own flourishing: we all rely on the help that others give us, and they in turn cannot give of their best to us if they are hampered by illness or disability. Nor, *pari passu*, can we help them to the full if we ourselves are hindered by the lack of necessary medical care. And there is an explicitly moral dimension to all of this as well. We cannot realize our potential to be good citizens or measure up to the moral obligations that society places on us if we are physically and mentally disabled in ways that could be corrected through proper medical care.

Health care, then, is endowed with moral qualities. If appropriate care is a necessary precondition for people to 'flourish' in their personal and social lives, then there must be a moral obligation to ensure that it is allocated fairly. For some to get more or better care than others for arbitrary or preferential reasons is socially unjust and morally indefensible. If health care resources are inadequate to allow everyone to 'flourish' to the highest possible degree, then they must be allocated in a way that gives everyone an equal crack at the whip. This, at heart, is the moral justification for the equitable allocation of health care, and for Doyal it is the reason why allocatory mechanisms based on cost-benefit studies or on publicly articulated preferences are morally flawed.

Allocation within, not between, different categories of treatment

But what would a morally justifiable structure of health care look like? How can Daniels' and Doyal's concern with the fair distribution of care be built into a complex health care system like the NHS? Doyal does not shirk the question. It could be done, he argues, by bringing the system into conformity with seven key principles. The first and most important is that a fair distribution of care would be within, rather than between, different categories of treatment. When difficult choices have to be made, the squeeze should be felt evenly among people needing all kinds of treatment. If we are to ration care fairly, the axe should not fall wholly or disproportionately on some treatments while others survive largely unscathed. To do so would be unjust to those who needed the treatments that happened to be in the axeman's sights.

Suppose, for example, that we could measure the proportion of people in a population needing treatment over a defined period of time for, say, heart disease, kidney disease, mental illness, and so forth. We could then, in principle, aggregate all these needs and multiply them by the unit cost of treating a typical case. The resultant sum would, naturally, be greater than the total budget available to the health care system, and some treatments would have to be provided at less than the volume indicated by the assessed need for them. But, Doyal argues, any such shortfalls should be spread evenly over *all* the categories of treatment, not focused disproportionately on some of them. If, for instance, the aggregate cost of meeting everyone's needs for care was 50 per cent greater than the available budget, then every treatment should be provided at 50 per cent of the demand for it. To do otherwise, Doyal asserts, would be to brand those suffering from some kinds of illnesses and disabilities (particularly those which lack clinical glamour or which carry overtones of shame and blame) as less deserving than others of the chance to 'flourish'. It would be morally indefensible.

Priorities within each category of need

Even if Doyal's first principle is observed, the question remains of how patients are to be selected for treatment within each category of need. How are those patients who *are* be treated within the available budget for each category of need to be distinguished from those who are *not*? Doyal's answer, logically, is that the priority accorded to each patient should be proportional to the threat that their illness or disability poses to their capacity to 'flourish'. This is the familiar principle of relative need: the greater the need for care (measured in terms of the severity of the threat to flourishing that the lack of care would pose), the higher should be the priority. Thus, top priority should be given to needs that threaten life, then to those that pose the risk of serious and irreversible disability, and so on. At the bottom of the range of urgency would be the familiar treatments that patients may want but do not really need: cosmetic surgery, the removal of benign lumps and bumps, and so on. The principle could be effected, Doyal proposes, through the use of triage in managing hospital waiting lists. To prioritize patients who are waiting to be treated in terms of the clinical urgency of their conditions, and then to treat them in that order, is to group them into morally similar divisions and to manage them in an equitable way.

Randomization as the last resort

Even to have followed Doyal's first two principles may not be to remove the need for further choices. Budgets for the management of some conditions in some localities may still be inadequate to allow all those in the same categories of need to be treated equally. How are further choices to be made between them? The answer, Doyal argues, must lie in randomization: if choices can no longer be made for reasons that are consciously articulated and morally defensible, then fairness requires a resort to some form of lottery. Such choices should certainly not be made according to the predilection of the doctors or the clinical challenge of a particular case. How randomization may feasibly be achieved is far from easy to imagine; but Doyal points out that waiting lists in fact allow for this because of the random time at which illness often strikes. Serious illness, in particular, is part of the 'lottery of life'. Provided the lists are actively managed along the lines of clinical triage (Doyal's second principle), then the ordering of patients *within* each category of severity will, effectively, be random. Where further choices have to be made beyond those mandated by the first two principles, all that needs to be done is to admit patients from each category in the order in which they entered the list.

Other preconditions

Doyal's final four principles are more in the nature of preconditions that the system must meet in order to gain a moral kitemark; and they are ones that we have already encountered. Scarce resources should not be spent on treatments that have been shown to be ineffective; people's chances of getting the care they need should never be influenced by their lifestyles; issues about the allocation of scarce resources for health care should be debated openly, explicitly and rationally and should not be hijacked for political reasons; and the views of the public should be heeded but not necessarily followed by those who manage the system. With all of these structures in place, Doyal contends, a health care system would be capable of making fair and morally defensible choices about the allocation of scarce resources. And, to the extent that his arguments are accepted, they would refute the contention of the House of Commons Health Committee in 1995 that there is no morally correct way of setting priorities. But even if they were to be accepted, is it possible to imagine that Doyal's principles could be implemented in the real world? His formulation certainly takes us closer to reality than Daniels'; but is it close enough to be practicable?

Applications

The centrality of need

The arguments of Rawls, Daniels and Doyal have in common the requirement that the structures and organizations of health care cannot be left to chance or interest: they must be planned and implemented in ways that can give embodiment to the principles of justice that each is seeking to achieve. The evidence that such conscious planning is being done, or even that it could be done, is patchy and impressionistic.

In their different ways, all three hold the notion of need to be central to their understanding of a just system. Rawls is concerned particularly with the needs of the least advantaged, Daniels with those that relate most closely to our capacity to achieve our lifetime goals and aspirations, and Doyal with those that must be tackled with the greatest urgency if we are to 'flourish' to the best of our abilities. As a generality, the culture of health care systems (particularly those which are centrally funded and politically driven) does reflect, to a greater or lesser degree, the importance of relative need in the way resources are rationed. No system openly dismisses the relevance of need in the ordering of people's claims, and all of them probably reflect the principles of triage in the way they work. In the NHS, high priority is almost always given to patients faced with a life-threatening emergency and to those whose conditions may give rise to permanent disability unless they are treated forthwith. Indeed, an increasing share of the work of the NHS has for several years been dominated by emergency work of one kind or another, almost at times to the neglect of patients with elective but nevertheless (to them) distressing conditions (Houghton and Hopkins, 1996).

Yet a general cultural acceptance of the importance of relative need in the just disposition of services is not quite enough. The formulations of Daniels and Doyal, in particular, require the principle to be built into the anatomy as well as the culture of the system. To implement Daniels' scheme, for example, the full spectrum of medical needs would first have to be fractionated according to the degree of adverse impact that each category of unmet need might have upon people's opportunities for 'species-typical normal functioning'; and health care systems would then have to be structured in a way that gave priority to each category in proportion to its degree of adverse impact. The political, managerial and intellectual obstacles of doing this are daunting, to say the least. According to what principles is the spectrum of need to be fractionated? Whose judgments are to be paramount when views collide? And where would be the humanity in a health care system that embodied such an approach, even if it were intellectually conceivable? Where, we might ask, are individual variations in all of this? Where is the scope for compassion? What becomes of clinical judgment? How are doctors to fulfil the ethical obligation of acting always in the best interest of their patients?

By contrast, the application of Doyal's vision of a just distribution is rather easier to imagine, not least because he goes much farther than

Daniels (and certainly than Rawls) in spelling out its implications. At the very least, we can begin to perceive the extent to which his major principles may *not* be reflected in the NHS, uncertain though we may be of the precise extent to which they are. His first principle, for example, is that rationing should occur within rather than between different categories of treatment. Such a principle has, for sure, never been formally accepted in the NHS and there is little firm evidence even of its informal salience in the minds of the politicians and planners. When the squeeze is on, those with the greatest degree of political muscle have invariably received the largest shares of the cake. For all the rhetoric of the years about the need to protect and nurture the 'priority' or 'Cinderella' services – those for elderly people and patients with mental illness and learning disabilities – such services have done consistently less well than those which are championed by patrons in positions of political power. Yet Doyal is surely right in arguing that the 'Cinderella' services can be just as vital to people's 'flourishing', if not more so, than heroic surgical interventions in their hearts, brains and abdomens; and if this is so, then there is a considered moral case for treating them no more but certainly no less generously than the glamorous specialities when the chips are down.

Doyal's second and third conditions affect the ways in which individuals are selected for treatment within each category of need. Priority should, he claims, be given in proportion to the threat that patients face to their capacity to 'flourish'; and when all such possibilities for triage have been exhausted, resort should be had to lottery. Much of this approach is probably reflected in the NHS through the active management of waiting lists by clinicians with a properly informed sense of social justice and a detailed understanding of their patients' conditions. As the 'stories' in Chapter 6 attest, the principles of triage do affect the order in which patients are selected for treatment. Yet there is no formal requirement to build such an approach into the anatomy of the system, and much depends upon local traditions and customs and the judgments of individual clinicians. Justice, as a systemic property, is subjugated to (or, rather, is expected to be effected through) clinical autonomy; and sometimes it seemingly fails to work.

The evidence of such failure is, for obvious reasons, difficult to find, but the veil has occasionally been lifted by knowledgeable commentators. One such is Yates (1995). Whether his conclusions are fair is not for the general observer to judge; but to the extent that they are, they are unquestionably forceful and disturbing. Yates' central concern is with the encroachment of the private work of surgeons on their capacity to deal fairly with their NHS patients. His principal conclusion is that:

those who cannot afford to pay for their treatment wait longer to get their treatment, get treated less frequently, are less likely to be operated on by a consultant and suffer greater levels of illness. The insured and the wealthy get treated more quickly, have more than their fair share of operations, are more likely to be operated on by a consultant and are likely to have lower levels of illness . . .

One-tenth of (NHS) patients receive one-fifth of the planned operations that our surgeons undertake, and a small but increasing proportion of our surgeons are now carrying out more than half their work in the private sector . . . (*op. cit.*, pp. 139–40)

Echoes of the veracity of such a claim are to be heard in the consultants' 'stories' in Chapter 6. Yates claims, moreover, that such failures are structural in origin.

There is neither an adequate consultant contract nor a monitoring mechanism in place to identify any abuse. The NHS does not know where its key employees are during the working day, nor has it any idea of the actual amount of work undertaken by any individual surgeon. Surgeons have too much scope to neglect the NHS in favour of their private work, and at the same time we find hugely different waiting times to see the same surgeon in the two competing sectors. (*op. cit.*, p. 141)

It scarcely requires the kind of analysis offered by Doyal to perceive the injustice that may result from the absence of systemic checks and balances on the way the waiting list is managed.

The way forward – a prototype?

Perhaps the closest example of the systemic approach to justice demanded by Daniels and Doyal is furnished by the report of the Dunning Committee, appointed by the Dutch government in 1990 to advise on the selection of national health care priorities (Dunning, 1992). When, early in their deliberations, the Committee's instinctive preference for some form of rationing by exclusion was frustrated by their government's reluctance to go down this particular path, they turned their attention instead to a 'screening' approach towards the prioritization of services. The result became known as the 'Dunning filters' – an iterative approach in which services or treatments are required to satisfy a progressive set of conditions in order to be included as priority services funded through the social insurance mechanism.

The first condition is communitarian: is the service necessary from the community point of view? To count as necessary, a service has to satisfy the Daniels-like criterion of adding to people's capacity for normal functioning. It was this consideration that enabled the Committee to give a high priority not only to the chronically sick, the elderly and the mentally ill but also to those facing life-threatening conditions. The next two conflated conditions, reflective of Doyal's fourth principle, are evaluative: has the service been demonstrated to be both effective and efficient, using such emerging procedures as evidence-based medicine and technology assessment? An element of judgment is plainly required in the severity with which these two conditions can be applied: too strict an application will jeopardize many services and treatments in daily use. The final criterion is personal necessity: is the service of sufficient importance to justify the expenditure of public money, or is it something akin to a luxury that people could reasonably be expected to provide for themselves? Dental care, homeopathic medicines, liposuction and sub-fertility treatment are examples of services which may be vulnerable to this criterion.

The Dunning Committee took the view that services and treatments which met all four criteria within reasonable limits should form the basic package of care funded by the Dutch government. That a service scored well on some abstract indicator of cost-benefit ratio, or was supported by public opinion, would *not* suffice unless it also passed the screening filters. Within the basic package, the Committee saw no further need for choice (of the kind, for example, envisaged by Doyal in his second and third principles): all services and treatments that made the final cut would be comprehensively available to all who required them. Any future reductions in the availability of real resources would be met not by instituting lotteries within the package but by ousting the least justifiable services from it.

A systemic approach to priorities of this kind might go some way towards meeting the concerns raised by Daniels and Doyal. Structural elements would be built into the anatomy of the health care system which would treat people equally (if not equitably) in their quest for care. If enforceable, it would also avoid the gross inequalities highlighted by Yates (1995) that can result from the idiosyncratic or self-serving management of waiting lists. Yet little happened in the immediate wake of the report (Honigsbaum, Holmström and Calltorp, 1997). It received a hostile reception from the civil servants in the Dutch Ministry of Health, and the politicians had difficulty grasping the nettle of choice. The Dunning philosophy became a symbol for doctors in their day-to-day work rather than an integral part of the structural fabric of health care. As always, it proved easier to develop guidelines than to bring about a structural change.

Yet all was seemingly not lost: parts of the Dunning Report began to be implemented in 1994 upon the appointment as Minister of Health, Welfare and Sport of an academic physician (Professor Els Borst-Eilers), whose own work had earlier influenced the thinking of the Dunning Committee (Spanjer, 1995). By 1995 dental care and physiotherapy had been dropped from the basic package for failing the Dunning filters and an evidence-based approach to medicine was receiving ministerial support. Whether the Dutch experience will demonstrate the practicability of long-term structural change in the name of justice will remain to be seen.

A dissenting voice: Nozick's entitlement theory of justice

Before leaving the structures of health care rationing and moving on to their processes, a dissenting note must be sounded, if only for the sake of even-handedness. The arguments of Rawls, Daniels and Doyal seem almost to take for granted the acceptability of using the power of the state to bring about a distribution of resources that is seen, on whatever criteria, to be a just one. There is, however, a strong tradition in political thought which cautions against the uncritical acceptance of such an assumption. It is a tradition which raises awkward questions not only about the meaning that is attached to the notion of a just distribution but also about the price that must be paid, usually in terms of encroachments upon individual liberties, to achieve it. For those who stand in this tradition, liberty cannot always and unquestioningly be sacrificed at the twin altars of welfare and equality. In the historical slipstream of the tradition are Locke and Mill; in the near-contemporary vanguard is the American philosopher Nozick, whose work seeks to define the minimal level to which the ethical state may go in involving itself in the lives of citizens without unjustifiably violating their rights (Nozick, 1974).

Just entitlements to possession

Within the notion of the ethical state as the 'minimal state', Nozick, like Rawls before him, seeks to build a theory of distributive justice. Described as the 'entitlement theory of justice', it holds, with striking simplicity, that any distribution is just if everyone is properly entitled to whatever portion of the bounty they are holding (*op. cit.*, pp. 150–1). If they are *not* so entitled, then the distribution is an unjust one. The bounty may be land, money, goods, services, health care, or whatever. A person's holding is just if either of two conditions is met: that the holding was justly acquired in the first place (the principle of 'justice in holdings') or that it was freely bestowed by another person who was entitled to hold it (the principle of 'justice in transfer'). It is a matter of common observation, Nozick argues, that many of the things which people actually hold have been acquired only through the violation of one or other of these two principles. 'Some people steal from others, or defraud them, or enslave them, seizing their product and preventing them from living as they choose, or forcibly exclude others from competing in exchanges' (*op. cit.*, p. 152). Whenever holdings have been acquired through unjust means of this sort, the resulting distribution is itself unjust and can properly be corrected through coercive action by the state (the 'principle of rectification'). But these are the only circumstances which can justify such coercive action.

Historical entitlement and patterned distributions

Central to Nozick's entitlement theory of justice is the idea that a just distribution must be judged not on the share-out of goods that can be observed at a particular moment in time, but on the processes through which it has been effected. It is, strikingly, a theory about history. It asks not about the justice (as Nozick defines it) of a given distribution of goods at a frozen moment of time, but about the justice of the means through which people acquired their holdings in the first place. Of course, this raises all manner of practical difficulties which Nozick does not try to evade. How far back do we have to go in order to wipe clean the slate of unjust acquisitions from the past? What obligations do those who have perpetrated past injustices have towards those whom they have wronged? Is the current generation liable for the injustices of its ancestors?

But whatever the practical difficulties, the historical core of the entitlement theory of justice is theoretically important because of its dramatic counterpoise to other, more popular, theories of distributional justice which ask no such historical questions. These theories, Nozick points out, are concerned only with what he calls 'end-result' or 'end-state' principles (*op. cit.*, p. 155). What matters for such theories is the justice of the *achieved* distribution, not the justice of the way it came about. Thus, for example, those who would see a just distribution of health care as one in which people's access to care was proportional to their need for it (and nothing else) would be interested only in the pattern, not its provenance. Nozick calls such distributions 'patterned distributions', and they are to be distinguished from distributions that result from an entitlement of holding.

Nozick invites us to consider, as an example, the category of distributional justice that is implied in the Aristotelian assertion that 'what is just in distribution must be according to merit in some sense' (see Chapter 2). It does not matter, for the purpose of the argument, what particular formulation of 'merit' is used. It might be need, it might be social or economic usefulness, it might be age – it doesn't matter. What does matter is that the resultant conception of a just distribution will be a *patterned* one: it will be one that corresponds to a pre-determined set of criteria that are judged to be morally relevant. Almost every suggested principle of distributional justice, Nozick argues, is patterned in this fashion: 'to each according to his moral merit, or needs, or marginal product, or how hard he tries, or the weighted sum of the foregoing, and so on' (*op. cit.*, pp. 156–7).

The entitlement theory of justice, by contrast, does *not* depend upon the achievement of a patterned distribution. People may justly acquire their holdings through many sources that conform to no pre-set patterns of justice at all: through their labour, through gambling or chance, through the earnings of a mate, through returns on investments, through gifts from friends, relatives and charities, and so on. Conversely, people may justly dispose of their holdings in all sorts of ways, including, if they so wish, gifts and charitable donations. Although it will, of course, be possible to perceive some common strands running through the acquisitions and disposals that people voluntarily make, the distribution which can be observed at any point in time is 'random with respect to any pattern . . . The process whereby the set of holdings is generated will be intelligible, but the set of holdings . . . that results from the process will be unpatterned' (*op. cit.*, pp. 157–8).

State power and patterned distributions

The next step in Nozick's argument suggests that, because patterned distributions would not arise in a society in which people's holdings were constrained *solely* by the entitlement theory of justice, such patterns can be maintained only through the continuous use of state power to interfere in the ways that people acquire and dispose of their just holdings. A patterned distribution – say, of health care – that is commonly seen as fair does not usually arise naturally, though it might do so in the unlikely event that everyone *freely* chose to acquire and dispose of their holdings in accordance with such a pattern. In this exceptional case, Nozick would recognize the allocation to be just *not* because it conformed to a prescribed pattern of fairness but because it resulted naturally from the free choices that people made about acquiring and disposing of their holdings. But such an exceptional case is simply that – exceptional. It is at this point, of course, that Nozick finds himself in explicit conflict with Rawls. Whereas Rawls relies on the conclusion that rational people will limit their tolerance of inequality to that which gives the best return to those who are least advantaged, Nozick replies that this is not how the world is. It is, he concedes, understandable that those who find themselves at the bottom of any pile should agree to having less than those at the top *if* this is the only way of improving their absolute position, but why should those at the top voluntarily limit the amount they receive *simply* in order to maximize the position of those at the bottom? Nozick dismisses the assumption that they would do so cheerfully and uncomplainingly as so much nerve (*op. cit.*, p. 195).

No, people do not freely arrange their holdings in patterned ways – certainly not those which correspond to predetermined notions of allocatory justice. It follows, then, that such patterns can be maintained *only* at the expense of violating the entitlement theory of justice, for they require the state to take away some of the holdings that people have justly acquired and give them to others. Such transfers are, by the definitions of Nozick's theory, unjust transfers because they do not result from the voluntary disposal of holdings by those who have a proper entitlement to them. As Nozick expresses the nub of the matter:

> no end-state principle or distributional pattern principle of justice can be continuously realised without continuous interference into people's lives . . . To maintain a pattern one must either continuously interfere to stop people from transferring resources as they wish to, or continually interfere to take from some persons resources that others for some reason choose to transfer to them. (*op. cit.*, p. 163)

This, Nozick claims, is simply a price too high. To interfere in people's lives in this way is to make unjustifiable encroachments upon their personal liberties. Liberties are best protected by the 'minimal state' – that is, a state which does little more than to protect people against force, theft and fraud and enforce the contracts into which they freely enter (*op. cit.*, p. ix). There is no room in such a state for coercive action either to take things from people (in the form of, say, taxes) that they would not freely dispose of in this way or to give things to people (in the form of, say, services) that others would not freely transfer to them. In plain language, any attempt to use the power of the state for redistributive ends is morally unjustified because it is bound to violate the way that

people would freely choose to acquire and dispose of their own holdings.

Nozick in perspective

What Nozick offers us is a morally principled counter-argument to the
core assumptions of Rawls, Daniels and Doyal. Their structures depend
in varying ways and to varying degrees upon the legitimacy of the state
– either directly through action in the public sector or indirectly through
regulations enforced upon the private sector – to bring about distributional patterns of health care that are judged to be 'fair' or 'just' in
relation to some predetermined criteria. For those who see the world as
Nozick does, the claimed morality of the distribution is, so to speak,
discounted by the higher-order immorality of the method by which it
has been brought about. To seek to allocate health care in proportion to
people's needs for it is, quite simply, morally unjustified if the price of
doing so is the violation of people's rights to acquire and dispose of their
justly held assets in ways of their own choosing.

Nozick's arguments about the structural requirements of a just society
constitute an important corrective to the conventional ethic of redistribution which permeates most of the liberal debate about health care
rationing. Whether we choose to take seriously his notion of the minimal
state as the ethical state must, in the final analysis, depend upon our own
political values. Even if his analysis is correct, we may feel that a degree
of violation of personal liberty *is* an acceptable price to pay for social
action that will improve the lot of the least advantaged, particularly if it
is regulated by a democratically elected government. Yet to say this is to
reveal a value which, ultimately, can be neither defended nor attacked.
The extent to which we are prepared to see the structures of the state used
to bring about a distribution of health care resources in favour of those
who are judged to have the strongest moral claims upon them is a
judgment that we each must make for ourselves.

4

Ethics and the processes of health care rationing

The challenge of process

The arguments of Rawls, Daniels and Doyal about the just distribution of resources have implications for health care at an institutional level: their insights are to be applied, to the extent that they can be, through the ways in which health care services are structured and organized. Yet as Chapter 3 suggested, these notions of distributive justice are expounded at a sufficiently high level of generality to make their translation from drawing board to building site a difficult one. To expect a country's health care system to conform to the architectural requirements articulated by, for example, Doyal, is to assume a degree of political and managerial control over the system, and a level of rational capacity within it, that might be seen, quite simply, as wishful thinking. As the 'stories' in Chapter 6 reveal, the rationing choices that are made at the front lines of the NHS are largely reactive, haphazard and unplanned.

This is neither to dismiss the force of the argument nor to abandon all attempts at creating a fairer structure; but it is to recognize that, in the medium term at least, the dream of architectural justice must be complemented, supplemented or replaced by a more practical focus on the way things are done. Not only must the *structures* of services be morally acceptable, so too must their *processes*. If a fair system of rationing is too elusive a concept to be captured by the institutional architecture, it may at least be reflected in the practices and procedures of those who work within it. It is something that must be *done*. To ask whether a particular distribution of public resources is or is not fair is fruitless. All that can sensibly be expected is that the decisions about the share-out should be reasonable. They should be 'publicly defensible on grounds that most people would regard as . . . relevant and fair' (Klein, 1998, p. 959). In the rather pessimistic formulation of Honigsbaum, Holmström and Calltorp (1997), 'the most that can be hoped is that it [priority setting] will be done in a way that is seen to be fair' (p. 115).

Broadly speaking, ideas about the moral acceptability of health care processes divide into two main groups: those that deal with the institutional processes of policy formulation and administration and those that relate to the more personal processes of clinical care. The distinction is by no means hard-and-fast, and important areas of overlap occur; but it suffices to give shape to the chapter. We begin with the institutional processes.

Responsive and responsible government

Responsive government

In his analysis of the morality of institutional processes, Weale (1990) draws a distinction between two contrasting styles of democratic government: responsive and responsible. The responsive style is one in which governments and their agencies try to provide the things that people want to have. The public's perceptions of its wants are notified mainly, though never exclusively, through the voting system, and elections between competing parties are fought mainly on the menu that each one offers. 'Vote for our party and we will give you what you want.' The responsible style of government, by contrast, is one in which political leaders are trying not merely to give the people what they *expressly* want but also to reason with them about the things they *ought* to want. Through discussion and dialogue, governments which operate in this fashion are trying to persuade the electorate, perhaps against their expressed wishes, that a particular course of action is the right one for the nation as a whole.

Weale argues that, although the responsive style of government is deeply embedded in western democratic traditions, it is a poor model for the way in which governments ought to be making decisions about the supply and allocation of health care resources. Although a particular voting system may show the broad sum of money that people wish to see expended on health care (and perhaps also an indication of how that money is to be distributed among different health care programmes), many electors' wishes will be swallowed up in the general trend of voting. A kind of average preference will be expressed (though different voting mechanisms will yield different averages); and whichever mechanism is adopted, many individuals will find their personal preferences ignored. In contrast to the majority views, they may wish to see either more or less money spent on the NHS and they may want a different balance of spending between alternative programmes.

Responsible government

Responsible government, on the other hand, sees its task as that of justifying a course of action which it judges to be right rather than sticking votes together in a particular way. Its authority comes from its ability to convince and persuade the electorate, and it is accountable for what it does. Accountability may take the form of explaining what the government has done in the light of what was promised, or, more profoundly, it may require the government and its agencies to expound and justify a chosen course of action and the ends to which it is directed.

Weale suggests that accountability of this kind requires a number of conditions to be met. Firstly, the decisions that are taken should be justified in an appropriate public forum. If this is done, then covert or partisan influences that might otherwise act against the public interest are likely to be squashed. It would, for example, be difficult for a fully accountable government to exempt a particular industry or sport from a general policy about health (such as the control of tobacco advertising) simply because that industry or sport had donated money to its political party. Secondly, the decisions that are taken should be broadly consistent with the prevailing political values of the society. The means by which the ends are to be attained must be in tune with the ways in which things are normally done in that society. And thirdly, since the essential task of a responsible government is to persuade and convince, it must treat each issue honestly and openly. A public dialogue between government and people in which essential items of information are withheld, or vested interests are concealed, is unlikely to engage the trust and the commitment of the electorate.

Responsible government and health care rationing

Weale's application of his notion of responsible government to the allocation of public resources for health care yields some demanding insights for Ministers and managers. Open, public and honest decision-making would require a British government to specify the standards and quality of care that could be produced from the resources it gave each year to the NHS; and if the gaze of professional and public scrutiny were to reveal the impossibility of attaining such standards, then either additional funds would have to be found or the standards revised. The public may not like the outcome, but it would have been reached through morally defensible means. Moreover, to the extent that the government's funding of the NHS fell short of providing effective care of a specified standard for all who could benefit from it, ministers would have to explain and justify the services most likely to feel the pinch – though to do so would, of course, run counter to the politician's instinct never to be explicit about bad news. Is it too surprising that Ministers, particularly those positioned more or less to the left of the political centre, are all too willing to aver that 'there is no such thing as rationing'?

Weale is careful to stress that responsible government would not eliminate the need to choose priorities: it would merely require the government to explain and justify how the choice had been made. It would *not* be acceptable for a government to evade responsibility for its choices either by pretending that no such choices were necessary or by claiming that more could be provided than its funding policy allowed. There is an obvious parallel with the mechanism of insurance: insurers have to state, with a good deal of precision, the benefits that will and will not be covered by a specified premium. It would be morally irresponsible for an insurer to take the premium without articulating the benefits that the policy-holder could expect and the circumstances under which he could expect them. Why should it be any different with government – even if what it collects are taxes rather than premiums? And wherein lies the morality of government insisting that doctors should increasingly be called to account for the quality of their work through clinical audit and other such measures, while evading a similar accountability itself? 'There is', Weale asserts, 'something essentially unsatisfactory about a service which for most people is a monopoly supplier of what is, sometimes literally, a life-saving resource which remains free to determine whether treatment should be withheld in particular cases and which does not have to defend legally the resource decisions that are made' (*op. cit.*, p. 127).

Of course, all democratic governments are, to some degree, open and accountable to the people they represent and serve. Weale's requirements for a responsible approach to health care rationing do, however, go some way beyond the point at which most governments and their agents are comfortable in their ways of working. British governments, for example, have never spelt out the volume and quality of care that can be afforded from the annual budget they provide for the NHS, nor have they ever indicated the increases or decreases in volume or quality that would follow from an expansion or contraction of the budget. Instead, the central selection of priorities has been a combination of guidelines, exhortation and obfuscation, leaving it largely to the coal-face workers to jiggle a quart of services from a pint pot of resources. British citizens are entitled to use the NHS, but they have never had many justiciable guarantees about the particular services they can expect to receive when they are ill (Newdick, 1995). Nor is the problem unique to the NHS: similar lacunae have given rise to concern elsewhere. The 1996 report of the Danish Council of Ethics, for example, found serious faults in the allocatory processes in Denmark, observing that there was 'no long term planning, allocation decisions were made in a piecemeal way, and many of the decisions were made by processes that were opaque to the general public' (Holm, 1998, p. 1001).

A prototype of responsible government? — the cases of Oregon and New Zealand

The Oregon experiment

There have, nevertheless, been signs in recent years of central and local governments moving a little closer to the more open and responsible mode that Weale describes. One such example is the American State of Oregon (Kitzhaber, 1993), whose attempt through its Health Services Commission to define the treatments that would and would not be available through the Medicaid programme in the State has already been described (Chapter 1). Not only does the outcome of the so-called Oregon experiment accord with Weale's requirement for transparency in the identification of services that will (and will not) be available through publicly funded systems of health care, the manner in which it was arrived at was, at least initially, honest and open. In a conscious attempt to ensure that its decisions resonated with public values, the Commission went to unusual lengths to allow the public to have their say — certainly beyond the outreach process required by the State legislature (Dixon and Welch, 1991).

First, the views of the public were sought through telephone surveys about the relative undesirability of different disabling conditions. Next, a series of 47 town hall meetings were held to elicit the values that people attached to different kinds of health care activity such as the treatment of addictions and the care of people with fatal and incurable conditions. The meetings were arranged by Oregon Health Decisions, a grassroots bioethics organization set up to educate Oregonians about the health policy choices confronting the State. Finally, the rankings produced by the Commission were exposed to the public in a further series of meetings, allowing special cases to be pleaded by individuals and interest groups.

The tragedy of Oregon was that this innovative attempt at responsible government largely failed (Honigsbaum, Holmström and Calltorp, 1997). The average attendance at the 47 town hall meetings was only 22, and few of these were Medicaid patients who would be affected by the outcome. Most were health workers with their own professional interest in what was happening. Hence the views and values emerging from the meetings were not only biased, they were biased towards the providers rather than the recipients or payers of care. In the event, the Oregon Health Commissioners largely abandoned their principled approach to the identification of priorities in favour of a pragmatic stance that blended public and professional values with their own perceptions of a fair way forward.

The New Zealand experiment

A somewhat different set of actions was played out in New Zealand in the early 1990s, though the objective was not dissimilar to Oregon's (Hadorn and Holmes, 1997). In 1992 the New Zealand government set in hand a major overhaul of its health care system designed to provide a more intelligent set of planning processes. The aim, as in Oregon, was the development of a transparent and explicit statement of what people could expect from their health care system and why; but whereas the Oregon Health Commission proceeded by identifying treatments that would *not* be available under the Medicaid programme, the National Health Committee in New Zealand adopted the alternative approach of specifying the circumstances under which each treatment or service *would* be available. Initially five procedures were included, including cataract extraction, coronary artery bypass grafting, and hip and knee replacement; and for each a standardized set of assessment criteria was developed by professional advisory groups that took account of such variables as patients' pain and movement, their functional ability, and their social and occupational responsibilities. The idea was that patients who 'scored' above a certain number of points could be assured of getting timely and relevant treatment in a consistent and fair manner.

The process of identifying the criteria also carried echoes of the Oregon approach. Public hearings were held by the National Health Committee on each island, particularly to gauge the sentiment of people on such contentious issues as the inclusion of social factors (such as the care of dependants and the capacity to work) in the assessment criteria. A stratified random sample of the public was invited to the meetings, together with groups of patients suffering from the conditions under consideration. As in Oregon, the hearings failed to generate any clear-cut public values (Hadorn and Holmes, 1997, p. 190); but the process was judged to be socially and politically useful. Overall, the programme's objective of ensuring equity and consistency in the process of identifying priorities for the New Zealand health service seems to have been well received. An Auckland newspaper, the *Dominion*, described it as 'light years ahead of rationing surgery by making people wait indefinitely for it, and with marked regional variations' (*op. cit.*, p. 191); and a cardiologist described the programme as offering a fair, humane and consistent approach to surgery in contrast to the current rampant practices of 'manipulation by referring doctors, friends in high places, MPs' letters, just persistent nagging, and just slight exaggeration of symptoms' (*op. cit.*, p. 193).

Explicit and implicit criteria of rationing

Explicit criteria of rationing and the NHS

Weale's advocacy of responsible government, and the echoes that it finds in the Oregon and New Zealand experiments, opens up some important moral issues in rationing processes. Three, in particular, are discussed at some length in the literature: the desirability of explicit or implicit criteria of rationing; the proper involvement of the public in rationing decisions; and accountability for rationing choices.

A responsible approach to rationing, in the way that Weale has defined the term, would seem to require it to be open and explicit. If it is to act responsibly, a government cannot plot its course of action behind closed doors and then impose it upon an ignorant electorate: it must be done in ways that can be seen and understood. Explicit choices about priorities must be explained, justified and defended. People must know the principles which underpin their chances of getting the care they require, and they must be able to challenge and change them if they do not like them. The argument applies not only to first-order choices made by governments and their agencies about the allocation of resources between different services and programmes, but also to second-order choices about the selection of patients for treatment. If some patients are to wait longer than others for the treatment they need, or even to wait in vain, they should know exactly what it is about their circumstances that has led to their lower priority. They may not like their wait, but at least they will know why it has occurred.

As we saw in Chapter 1, some allocatory mechanisms offer precisely this kind of certain knowledge. In a freely operating private market for health care, those who get the worst kind of treatment, or none at all, are well aware of the reasons for their plight: they are unable or unwilling to pay the going rate. Third-party insurance, which is the means by which most people are able to pay for private health care, is usually very precise in the information it provides about the benefits that are available under each policy. Policy-holders know exactly where they stand. The same is true (though the language is different) under systems of rationing by entitlement. Military men in the eighteenth century knew the exact amount of food they would receive each day, and British civilians in World War II were similarly aware of the monthly rations they would receive for food, clothing and other essential goods (Chapter 1). It was above board. It was explicit.

Until recently, however, the NHS in the UK has rarely worked in such an explicit mode. If rationing processes in health care can be seen in terms of a spectrum of explicitness (Mechanic, 1977), then the British health care system has been located fairly well towards the implicit end. Few guarantees have been given about the circumstances under which people can be assured of care. Until they need an operation or require respite care or seek the services of a physiotherapist, people may have no more than an anecdotal awareness of the speed with which such services can be mobilized on their behalf, if at all, or the fullness of a service when it does arrive. And there are influential voices that approve of such fluidity. In the important case of Jaymee Bowen, the Master of the Rolls declared it to be 'totally unrealistic' for the Cambridge Health Authority to have to justify its decision not to fund Jaymee's referral to the Hammersmith Hospital (*The Times Law Report*, 1995). The authority was not required to explain its reasons publicly; it was sufficient that, having weighed up all the relevant factors and taken expert advice, the authority thought it right not to fund the referral. The Master of the Rolls declared himself unable to fault the procedure that the authority had gone through, and he accordingly found in its favour. Support for this view has come from high places in British medicine. Sir Raymond Hoffenberg, a former President of the Royal College of Physicians, declared in his Harveian Oration that 'if services are to be limited, I would rather see it done implicitly – unstated, unwritten, unacknowledged – in the curious and not inhumane way in which such matters are managed in the United Kingdom' (quoted in Smith, 1991b, p. 1562).

Such views appear to sit increasingly uncomfortably against the rapidly shifting cultures of public as well as private services. For all that the so-called new managerialism has imposed a weight of bureaucratic obligation on those who work in them, it has also elevated the status of those who use them. To redesignate patients as customers or clients may seem tedious or even patronizing; but it signals a change in the way they are to be treated by organizations. Customers have rights and expectations. They are paying for the goods and services they receive, even if indirectly as taxpayers, and they are entitled to know exactly what they are getting for their money. If something cannot be done, or cannot be done for a long time, then customers have a right to be told why. It is not sufficient for providers to hide behind the screen of managerial or clinical discretion.

The recent history of the NHS can be read, in part, as the history of movement from implicit to more open and explicit forms of rationing (Hunter, 1995). General practices now publish annual reports in which they explain their policies about appointments, out-of-hours care, and the services they do and do not offer. Patients' charters set target waiting times to see a consultant. Promises are made about the speedy access to specialist diagnosis for patients with suspected cancers. On the provider side, clinicians are coming under increasing pressure to explain and justify their decisions. National service frameworks will make much more explicit the range and quality of services that patients can expect (Department of Health, 1997a). The introduction of the NHS information superhighway will increase the ease with which people can find out what is happening. As more and more doors begin to open, the territory of hidden, implicit rationing will steadily shrink.

For the most part, such moves have been welcomed as part of the drive towards more open government. With a prescience of understanding and a choice of language that still seems remarkable, Enoch Powell in the mid-1960s anticipated the controversy that rationing in the NHS would arouse and placed himself on the side of openness (Powell, 1966). Reflecting on his earlier experiences as Minister of Health he concluded ('brutally', as he put it) not only that care in the NHS has to be rationed, but that the processes of rationing are inherently political in nature:

> The task is not made easier by the political convention that the existence of any rationing at all must be strenuously denied. The public are encouraged to believe that rationing in medical care was banished by the National Health Service, and that the very idea of rationing . . . is immoral and repugnant. Consequently when they, and the medical profession too, come face to face . . . with the various forms of rationing to which the National Health Service must resort, the usual result is bewilderment, frustration and irritation. (*op. cit.*, p. 38)

The only way to circumvent such bewilderment, Powell concluded, was political transparency about what was happening. 'The worst kind of rationing is that which is unacknowledged; for it is of the essence of a good rationing system to be intelligible and consciously accepted' (*op. cit.*, p. 38).

The moral case for explicit criteria of rationing

An overtly moral case for clarity in the rationing process, flowing logically from his notions about a just structure of health care (see Chapter 3), has been put by Doyal (1997a). The case rests in part upon a principled resistance to the unavoidable element of public deception to which implicit rationing inevitably gives rise. To deny people treatment while failing to explain the reason is at best to keep them deliberately in the dark and at worst to mislead them about the truth of a situation that could seriously affect their health and well-being. Such deception (the argument goes) is intrinsically wrong and should be contemplated only if it is clearly the lesser of two evils. Nor is it fair to those who have to conspire in the deception. 'It is not good enough', argues Maxwell, 'to place the distasteful and increasingly onerous task of rationing on the shoulders of the clinicians and tell them to close the gap between need and provision by trying ever harder' (Maxwell, 1995b, p. 943).

More positively, Doyal argues that the case for clarity rests also upon the clear moral principles on which the NHS was founded. They may be rather general in their content and fuzzy at their edges; but they do exist (Rivett, 1998, p. 30). The NHS was founded to provide care to those who need it most, regardless of race, wealth or creed. Its goal was the equal treatment of all in equal need, whoever they were and wherever they happened to live. It was designed to be egalitarian in purpose – to deal with all the people fairly. How, Doyal asks, can we cling to these principles while simultaneously denying people the right to know the manner in which they are being implemented and the extent to which they are succeeding? If we really believe that people's access to the NHS should be in proportion to their need for the care it provides, we must understand how such a precept is being translated into practice at both policy and clinical levels. And if the service is seriously striving towards such a goal, it must also reveal the information by which the people can judge its success. If a principled NHS means anything, it must mean an open and transparent dialogue between the government and the governed. How else can voters be expected to take an informed and intelligent interest in the governance of their communities? How else can they judge whether knowledgeable or clinically interesting patients are not being preferred to dull or clinically commonplace ones? How else can the bias of the street-level bureaucrat be monitored and corrected?

The moral case against explicit criteria of rationing

It is a powerful case; but not one that goes unopposed. The counter-argument in favour of what has so far been the traditional approach to rationing in the NHS has three main prongs. One is simply pragmatic: for all the high-minded talk about the principles of the NHS, the fact remains that it is a complex, multi-dimensional organization, embracing different professional and political interests, reflecting a plurality of cultures and moral values, and struggling in all its many parts to cope with the demands it faces from the resources it commands. As with any complex health care system, its goals are diverse and often conflicting: to treat disease, to maximize health, to meet people's needs and expecta-tions, to foster social equality and to nurture the community's sense of security (Holm, 1998). To expect such a many-headed hydra to speak with a single concerted moral voice is to bay for the moon. It may not even be wise: 'given the plurality of often conflicting values that can be brought to any discussion of priorities in health care, it is positively undesirable (as well as foolish) to search for some set of principles or techniques that will make our decisions for us: the idea of a machine for grinding out priorities is wrong' (Klein, 1993, p. 310). And in any case, real-life attempts to create such a machine, in almost every country where they have been made, have foundered on the rocks of political pluralism. Those with the authority to thrash out the necessary formulae have simply failed to do so. The stark reality is that we may have no realistic option other than to proceed along the implicit path we are already treading.

There are two other, rather more principled, arguments in favour of discretionary rationing. The first is that, on balance, it creates more human happiness than the alternative (Coast, 1997). Patients naturally do not like to be told that nothing can be done for them, or that they must wait rather longer than they had expected for the treatment they need; but the emotional impact of any such disappointment can, to a degree, be absorbed and deflected by those who give them the news (Sabin, 1998). As Aaron and Schwartz (1984) found, doctors may soften the blow by presenting it in medical terms (see Chapter 1). There is, they will say, regrettably little that can be done. Hard though that may be to bear, it is (the argument goes) less hard than the alternative of knowing that effective treatment is technically available but has been delayed or withheld for reasons of cost. The muffled discretionary approach fosters a more stable and trusting relationship between doctor and patient and it minimizes friction. The point is a moot one: some may see implicit rationing one way, others the other. Medical bad news is intrinsically unwelcome, but doctors are ethically obliged to be honest with patients who ask about their prognosis. Bad news that springs from economic rather than biological sources may be no different.

A second, and perhaps more persuasive, argument in favour of discretionary rationing is that of flexibility: it can respond sensitively to the heterogeneity of patients, doctors and treatments (Mechanic, 1995). It is an argument that fits more naturally into the clinical world of the doctor than the policy world of the bureaucrat. Diversity and uncertainty are part of the very stuff of medical practice: treatments that appear to work well for some patients under some circumstances may do little or nothing for others in different circumstances. Medical practice still retains its traditional elements of judgment and intuition, even in the midst of the surging tide of evidence-based care; and a measure of clinical discretion remains a patient's sure defence against a bureaucratic rule to which he may well be the exception. Thus, the rule may be that the removal of tattoos carries a low priority in the minds of politicians and managers; the reality may be that a fund-holding practice would see the cost to be justified in the particular case of the young woman whose promising career as a model (and whose good mental health) is placed in jeopardy by an artistic indiscretion of earlier years.

A responsible culture of medical practice, Mechanic argues, would be one in which doctors accepted responsibility for their stewardship of scarce resources, working within a common framework of understanding about best practice and cost-effective care. Patients are no longer to be understood as passive and grateful recipients of whatever the system chooses to give them. They are, rather, active collaborators in their own care, with views, tastes and preferences that have a rightful place in the matrix of decision-making about their care. No two patients are exactly the same. The more explicit become the rules about access and entitlement, the less the scope for bespoke decisions tailored to the needs of each patient. 'Implicit rationing', Mechanic argues, 'provides the flexibility to do so, whereas explicit mandates rigidify the alternatives through a superficial assessment of equity-efficiency trade offs' (*op. cit.*, p. 1658).

Public involvement in rationing decisions

The issue of public involvement

Similar moral dilemmas surround the proper involvement of the public in the rationing processes of the NHS. Weale's (1990) notion of responsible government seems clearly to imply a form of structured partnership between the elected and the electorate (see also Weale, 1995). It requires government neither to impose its own priorities on a passive citizenry nor slavishly to follow whatever tangle of preferences might emerge from any particular way of sampling public opinion. Responsible government is about listening to the voices of the people, informing them honestly of the issues and choices they are facing, and discussing with them the best ways forward. It is, of course, much easier to offer this as a principle than it is to suggest realistic ways in which it can be embodied: the experiences of other states and countries which have tried to make it work, most notably Oregon and New Zealand, are not entirely encouraging (Honigsbaum, Holmström and Calltorp, 1997; Hadorn and Holmes, 1997). But is the principle itself correct? Is it right that the views of ordinary citizens and patients, unconnected in any other way with the health care system and uninformed about its subtlety and complexity, should be accorded any weight at all in the rationing of public resources? Is the rationing process made more moral by their inclusion and would it be rendered less so by their exclusion?

Even to raise such a question might seem outrageous in these empowering times. The consumerist revolution sweeping through the corridors of private corporations and public services alike has elevated the users of the NHS from mere supplicants, gratefully receiving whatever care is given to them by a benign and generous cadre of officials, to customer-kings, demanding their rights and wanting to be heard. In 1992 the NHS Management Executive urged local health authorities to sample the views of the public on local purchasing issues (National Health Service Management Executive, 1992), and the Secretary of State later insisted that they 'must actively seek to encourage public participation in . . . establishing priorities and in making decisions based upon them' (Mihill, 1993, p. 2). It was an important milestone in the history of consumer participation in the NHS and one that much of the British press endorsed in the wake of the case of Jaymee Bowen. The *Guardian* insisted that 'the public must be involved'; the *Independent* that 'the only way forward is a more transparent and accountable NHS . . . in which ordinary people could play their part in setting priorities'; and the *Observer* that 'the ministry must . . . promote the structures which involve the public in the decision making' (quoted in Entwistle *et al.*, 1996, p. 100). Readers were apparently to draw the conclusion that 'the public' would not have denied a young child like Jaymee the chance of extending her life, however uncertain the treatment or whatever the cost.

The moral case against public involvement

Against the combined forces of the executive and the fourth estate, Doyal (1993, 1997b) has set out the principled case against the involvement of the public in rationing choices – or, more precisely, the limits of their proper involvement. It is a case that flows logically from his structured specification of a just health care system (see Chapter 3), and it is of a kind not unlike that by which he defends the explicit rationing of care. The case is, quite simply, that the 'moral foundations of the NHS are not up for democratic grabs' (Doyal, 1997b, p. 178). A morally defensible structure for the health care system can, Doyal maintains, be worked out from first principles: it is one which acknowledges that people's legitimate needs for health care are those which hinder their capacity to flourish fully as responsible citizens and in which the severity of their need is the only proper basis for discriminating among them. We do not need to consult the public about this, and if public opinion delivers a divergent pattern of priorities, then we should ignore it.

> The moral foundations of the NHS do not depend on a majority vote or individual preference for their moral coherence. Their justification starts and finishes with the quality of moral argument employed, along with the empirical evidence referred to in such an argument. It follows that principles of equality and fairness in the rationing of health care should not be open to change on any other basis. (*op. cit.*, p. 179)

In short, the public may not be trusted to deliver a just solution.

There is a certain amount of evidence to support Doyal's sceptical view of public opinion – provided, of course, that we accept the particular criteria of justice that he would have us accept and also that we can agree about the arguments by which they are derived. Publicly expressed priorities for health care rationing, insofar as we can know them from the limitations of the technologies by which they are garnered, can be inconsistent and may even be unashamedly partial. In general, the treatment of acute life-threatening conditions, particularly for children, stands higher in public favour than the promotion of good health or the long-term care of older people (Kneeshaw, 1997). More particularly, the first nationwide survey of public views about priorities in the NHS revealed attitudes and dispositions that were partially reflective of a preference for equity, but which also ran counter in certain respects to current ethical thinking (Bowling, 1996). Carried out among a randomly selected national sample of 2,005 people in Britain (with a response rate of 75 per cent and no great response bias), the interviews required the respondents to articulate the relative importance they would attach to 12 different service items chosen to span the range of activity in the NHS. The items included, for example, special care and pain relief for terminally ill people, screening and immunization services, surgery such as hip replacements to help people carry out their everyday tasks, intensive care for premature babies with only a slight chance of survival, and treatment for people over 75 with life-threatening illnesses. The attitudes of respondents to a number of options in the rationing process were also harvested.

Doyal's fear about the threat that democratic participation might pose to the moral foundations of the NHS is justified to some degree by the results of Bowling's survey. It would, for example, be difficult to say that the views expressed in the survey accorded entirely with the core principle of equal care for equal need – but then, the questions were not asked in a way that helped the respondents to think in such terms. And in any case, how can we know what people understand by 'equal need' without an altogether more probing form of enquiry than a structured interview, however well conducted it may be? That said, however, it seems clear from the results that the public are rather less responsive than Doyal would wish them to be to the idea that care should be rationed within rather than between services. Central to Doyal's formulation is the moral claim that, when difficult choices have to be made, the squeeze should be felt evenly among people needing all kinds of treatment. If we are to ration care fairly, the axe should not fall wholly or disproportionately on some treatments while others survive largely unscathed.

The public's preferences, to the extent that they were disclosed in Bowling's survey, were otherwise: her respondents seemed quite content to make just such a blanket choice. Overwhelmingly, for example, they favoured the treatment of children with life-threatening illness above that of old people *in similar situations of need*. Half of all the respondents in the survey placed the former in their top two priorities while only 5 per cent ranked the treatment of life-threatening conditions for the over-75s among their top two. Other attitudes revealed by the survey also sat uncomfortably with Doyal's formulation. More than two-fifths of the respondents agreed that people who contributed to their own illnesses (for example though smoking, obesity or excessive drinking) should have a lower priority than those with more prudent lifestyles: yet one of Doyal's preconditions of fairness (that people's chances of getting the care they need should not be dependent upon such considerations) is widely shared among contemporary ethicists. Or again, three-quarters of the respondents thought that the responsibility for health care rationing should rest with doctors rather than politicians or managers: yet micro-rationing at this level is always likely to offend Doyal's formal requirement that the substance and bases of rationing choices must always be explicit.

The moral case for public involvement

None of this is *necessarily* to say that the public is wrong or that their views should be set aside; but it is to say that the issue is, inescapably, a contested one. Doyal's position seems to require him always to set boundaries to the involvement of the public in the formal argument about distributional justice. Others are less sure. One such is Coote (1997). Her position is not dissimilar to that of Weale (1990). She first draws the familiar tripartite distinction between clinical decisions, executive decisions and political decisions which define the goals and values of the NHS. The first two domains, Coote concedes, are not ones in which the layman has much of a part to play: because members of the general public lack the technical expertise of the clinician and the manager, the system would collapse if they were to claim a say in such decisions. But decisions about the meaning and purpose of the NHS, including decisions about the just allocation of public resources, are different because they are rooted in the fundamentally political nature of the process. Deciding what is 'fair' is, at heart, a political activity and politics is about people. Thus, Coote envisages 'an open and mature relationship between ordinary citizens and decision makers' (*op. cit.*, p. 161), fostering and feeding the trust that is increasingly seen as a vital component in the management of public services. Trust is the key; but it is, Coote claims, eroding away and it can no longer be built on a platform of benign paternalism which 'claims to protect and provide but fails to consult or involve' (*op. cit.*, p. 162).

The weaker the mechanisms for public education and participation, the more contested become the rationing decisions which the service is forced to make. Public opinion is stirred over reports of people waiting hours for urgent treatment on trolleys in out-patient departments, or over visible evidence in their localities of the failures of community care for people with mental illness, precisely because the realities of the funding of the NHS and the choices they inevitably pose have never been explained to, and shared with, the people. Instead, they have been encouraged to believe that all things are possible even in the face of political promises to reduce the headline rate of taxation. The result, Coote contends, is a growing sense of injustice and insecurity. People have rarely had the chance to express their views about a just approach to health care – or even whether they want an avowedly just system at all. We know little of what the electorate thinks about the wisdom of a continuing commitment to Aneurin Bevan's grand vision of a comprehensive state service, meeting all their needs from the cradle to the grave. We know only in very general terms how far wage-earners are prepared to.go in trading off a comprehensive service against higher taxation. It is a matter of guesswork whether most people would share the principles of equity implicit in Rawls' or Daniels' or Doyal's notions of structural justice. By trusting the public's ability to understand and contribute to the complex dilemmas of choice, the decisions that have to be made will carry a valued measure of democratic legitimacy. It may be a risky strategy, but it is better than doing nothing.

Practical exercises in public involvement

So much for the theory. The practice is rather more difficult to envisage and engineer. Public opinion may be a powerful force when it is mobilized for a purpose, but if it is to function fairly it must be educated, led and moderated. Exercises in public consultation can all too easily collapse into overt civic self-interest – the 'not-in-my-back-yard' syndrome – when it comes to the siting of community care facilities for people with mental illness or learning difficulties, and the 'in-my-back-yard' syndrome when it comes to the siting of acute hospital services. Perhaps we should not be too surprised at this. Why should people not struggle to protect what they regard as the best interests of themselves and their communities? To do so is understandable, perhaps even moral. Why should they lift their eyes beyond their immediate horizons and try to understand that others may have even greater needs? Is it not expecting too much of humanity that it should take a dispassionate and disinterested position on abstract principles of social justice? Is not the assurance of justice a matter for governments and their agencies – if necessary in the teeth of public opposition?

Yet the voices of the optimists can be heard in all of this. It is, Coote (1997) contends, not only *necessary* for the public to be more involved than they are at present, it is also *possible* to take their views more directly into account in rationing decisions. Various methods, more or less tried and tested, are available and examples of good practice are to hand (National Health Service Management Executive, 1992; Murray *et al.*, 1994). Opinion polls, for example, are relatively cheap and flexible, but they do not foster dialogue and the views they garner are likely to be rather superficial and uninformed. Public meetings, as the experiences in Oregon and New Zealand affirm, appeal most to those who probably have the least at stake. Rather more promising are 'citizens' juries' of about a dozen people, chosen according to some notion of representativeness, which meet on a regular and prolonged basis to discuss particular issues that are put to them (Coote and Lenaghan, 1997). They have the time to become informed about each issue and they can contemplate it at some length. Where they have been tried, juries appear capable of delivering a reasoned set of views about the matter in hand. The difficulty, for health authorities, is knowing what to do with their verdicts. There is little point in creating such groups if their pronouncements are then ignored; but they may well deliver maverick opinions that run counter to existing policy or ethical opinion – and what then?

Just such an example has been reported from Somerset, where a citizens' jury (though it was actually called a focus group) was asked to consider the circumstances, if any, under which coronary bypass operations should be denied to cigarette smokers (Bowie, Richardson and Sykes, 1995). The issue was highlighted by the case of Harry Elphick in 1993, who was refused cardiac surgery following a heart attack until he had given up smoking (see Chapter 2). Ethical opinion in the wake of the case broadly favoured the view that patients whose behaviour may in some degree have caused their illness should not suffer discrimination on that ground alone. The Somerset jury, however, took a modified view of the matter, recommending that *second* bypass grafts should not be offered to smokers provided they had been duly advised the first time round. The recommendation was implemented by the health authority. Public opinion was heeded; but whether at the cost of a loss of moral integrity is precisely the issue at stake.

Accountability for rationing decisions

Political accountability

The issue of accountability for the rationing choices that have to be made in the NHS cannot easily be separated from those of openness and public participation. In Weale's (1990) vision of responsible government, accountability would be exercised within the ancient conventions of democratic politics (Day and Klein, 1987). In the Athenian state, those who ran the affairs of society were required regularly to explain and justify their conduct to the assembly of citizens; and if they failed to carry the confidence of the citizenry, they faced trial by jury. With the growing complexity and diversity of human society, direct accountability to the people became ever less feasible and was supplanted by a less direct accountability to representative assemblies. In England the power of

Parliament increased from Tudor times onwards, replacing the monarch as the primary locus of accountability at a national level. Councils of elected representatives did the same at a local level. Ministers and their Civil Servants (and their counterpart councillors and officers in local government) came increasingly to be held to account by each assembly for their stewardship of the powers delegated to them.

More recent accretions to the machinery of government (such as agencies, executives, ombudsmen and the like) have complicated the simple model of accountability to representative assemblies, but the principles and preconditions remain. Those who manage the affairs of society, in all its diversity and complexity, must be capable of being held to account for what they do. For accountability to work, however, the necessary linkages must be in place by which they can be required to explain and justify their behaviour to the representatives and can be admonished or removed by them if they are found wanting. And the representatives in their turn must be held accountable to the people, at the very least by submitting themselves periodically for election in open and fair ballots.

At a superficial level, such linkages work acceptably well in the UK. The House of Commons can and often does cross-examine Ministers about the running of their Departments, and the various Committees of the House do likewise with Civil Servants and their agents and officials. On certain topics, at least, the people are allowed a reasonably full glimpse of the issues. Less convincing, perhaps, is the capacity of the representatives to admonish or dismiss those whose behaviour fails to find favour. Ministers, for example, seem less inclined to resign nowadays than they used to be, seeking protection in recent years in the developing doctrine of cloven responsibility for policy and operations. If a high-profile prisoner escapes from a high-security jail, that is apparently a failure of operations for which the Director of the Prison Service must pay the price. It is not a failure of policy, for which, *if it were*, the Home Secretary would naturally do the decent thing and resign.

The linkages that are formally required for effective accountability are, in principle, more clearly in place in the NHS than in many other areas of public life or service. The constitutional position was hammered out in 1945–6 when the Labour government was preparing its legislation to take the public hospitals away from local government and place them under the control of non-elected regional boards and management committees (Webster, 1988, p. 84). 'Such bodies', wrote the then Minister of Health, Aneurin Bevan, in 1945, 'will be the agents (though, not, I hope, in any derogatory sense, the creatures) of my Department' (quoted in Day and Klein, 1987, p. 76). Bevan was clear that, although appointed through channels of professional representation and local patronage, the members of such bodies should be accountable to the Minister and through him to Parliament. If a bedpan was dropped on a hospital floor, he wanted the sound of it to echo through the Palace of Westminster.

The constitutional position has probably remained unchanged throughout the lifetime of the NHS in spite of the series of major structural reorganizations, begun in 1974, that have transformed the managerial face of the service. Technically, the directors of the health authorities and NHS trusts are the agents of the Secretary of State, appointed by and accountable to him through the NHS Executive. In principle, they can be dismissed if their behaviour fails to please. In practice, however, the clarity with which the links in the lengthening chain of public accountability can be seen and approved by the electorate has been clouded by an unresolved (and perhaps unresolvable) tension between the democratic centre and the unelected periphery. In area after area of public life, including the NHS, elected government is being replaced by appointed government. Those who are elected count for ever less while those who are appointed count for ever more, and they are increasingly able to work in ways that evade any effective form of democratic scrutiny (Weir and Hall, 1994, p. 44).

At the centre, Ministers fervently wish the NHS to succeed in the eyes of the electorate, for therein lie many votes. They are eager for local managers and executive directors to do their bidding whenever it suits their purposes, and they are all too ready to grab the credit for the good news while blaming the locals for the bad. The managers and executive directors, however, may see it rather differently: while obligated to implement whatever legislation has been passed by a democratically elected Parliament, their motives are shaped by additional considerations, among them the need to balance the competing desires and wishes of local pressure groups, to respond to the distinctive needs of their local populations, and to advance their own careers. Somewhere between the centre and the periphery is a largish hole into which effective accountability can all too easily tumble and be lost. If a health authority quietly drops a number of services from the menu of those which it provides through the NHS, in what sense can it be said to be accountable for its actions? If health authority members, in the name of rationalization, close or downgrade an acute hospital, thus reducing the quality or accessibility of care to those it serves, how can the community call them to justify their behaviour and admonish or remove them if they find it wanting? The constitutional position notwithstanding, there is often, in practice, a disturbing democratic deficit in the NHS that cannot be concealed behind cosmetic plans to heed the voices of the people (Pollock, 1992).

Professional accountability

The picture is further complicated by the pervasive factor of professional (particularly but not exclusively medical) autonomy, wafting like incense through the wards and boardrooms of the NHS. As members of a state-licensed monopoly, doctors have been among the most successful professions in protecting their freedom from managerial control and insisting upon their accountability only to their peers. Though employed by or (in the case of the GPs) contracted to the NHS, doctors in the UK cannot routinely be held to account for their clinical decisions either by their paymasters or by their patients, however much their decisions may shape the patterns of rationing to which their patients are exposed. A patient who feels unfairly discriminated against because of the way her doctor has chosen to treat her can find it all but impossible to call the doctor to account either personally or through the constitutional mechanisms of accountability in the NHS. Formal appeals are of course possible (Department of Health, 1994), but the service would simply collapse if even a minuscule proportion of the rationing decisions made by doctors were contested in this way.

Whether or not doctors are *effectively* accountable to their peers is also open to question. A formal accountability springs from their state licensure: doctors are registered by the statutorily founded General Medical Council (GMC) and can have their licence to practise withdrawn by it. Understandably, however, the GMC formally enquires into the activities of doctors only when there is a serious case to answer: it would be both impossible and intolerable for the Council to concern itself with the minutiae of day-to-day decisions that affect the allocation of care to patients. It has, in any case, been criticized by knowledgeable observers for its resemblance to an exclusive gentlemen's club, concerned as much with protecting the profession's power and status as safeguarding the interests of patients (Stacey, 1992). Yet neither does there appear to be any guarantee that less formal and more local systems of peer review can systematically protect patients from the behaviour of unjust, incompetent or maverick practitioners.

In 1998 the GMC found three Bristol doctors guilty of serious professional misconduct, removing the names of two of them from the register (*The Lancet*, 1998). The core charge was that the rates of operative and post-operative deaths among children upon whom they performed cardiac surgery were much higher than usual for such operations.

Evidence emerged in the course of the GMC's enquiry that the high deaths rates were known not only by their local colleagues but also by the Department of Health and the Royal College of Surgeons; yet nothing was done. Formal action was taken only when an anaesthetist finally 'blew the whistle' and paid the price for his intemperance by being forced to continue his career abroad. Of course, the charge of serious professional misconduct is altogether more grave than that of bias or injustice in the allocation of resources; but if professional accountability can fail in the former, what chance may there be for the latter? The linkages in the chain of accountability, as in the Bristol case, may be weak or even missing. As *The Lancet* commented,

> the picture that emerges . . . is one in which many professionals, from nurses in the operating theatre to government officials, were aware that there was a problem. Yet there was no clear chain of command and communication to ensure that the difficulties were remedied at the earliest possible point. If the organisations that regulate the medical profession do not put their heads together now and create a system to . . . deal with problems in clinical practice as they emerge, the Bristol story is bound to be retold elsewhere. (*op. cit.*, p. 1669)

Ethical codes of medical practice

The need for codes

The question of the accountability of doctors and other clinicians, not least for the rationing decisions in which they may be implicated, is being addressed increasingly within the context of ethical codes of medical practice (Hurwitz and Richardson, 1997). At most times and in most places, those who practise the healing arts have voluntarily placed themselves under corporate moral codes that govern their behaviour with those they treat. Such codes commonly oblige doctors to respect the integrity of their patients (autonomy), to do them good (beneficence), and never knowingly to cause them harm (non-maleficence) (Calman, 1997). Their well-spring is the notion of personhood. Patients are to be treated with respect and their interests are to be paramount not because of any merit or distinction they may possess, or because they are deserving of medical attention, or because of the clinical interest of their conditions, but simply because they are people. 'May I never see in the patient anything but a fellow creature in pain.' These words, attributed to the twelfth-century Spanish physician Maimonides, express the ideal towards which all medical intervention in the life of another person is directed (quoted in Porter, 1997, p. 101).

The content of codes

Moral aspirations of this kind have been codified in several texts. Best known, perhaps, is the Hippocratic Oath dating from around 400 BCE, requiring those who affirm it to ensure that their actions are 'for the benefit of my patients' and that they will abstain from 'whatever is deleterious and mischievous'. Though it is to be doubted whether Hippocrates actually set out to establish a system of moral values in medicine (Horner, 1996), the Hippocratic Oath has formed the bedrock of western medical ethics and is still used or administered in medical schools in the USA (Crawshaw, 1994) and the UK (Delamothe, 1994). More modern in its language and ideas is the Geneva Convention Code of Medical Ethics, adopted by the World Medical Association in 1949. It binds doctors to make the health of their patients their first consideration, to maintain the utmost respect for human life from the time of conception, and to prevent considerations of religion, nationality, race, party politics or social standing from intervening between duty and patient.

Lacking the moral imperative of a code, but probably more widely read in the UK than either the Hippocratic Oath or the Geneva Code, is the guidance on good medical practice from the General Medical Council (General Medical Council, 1995). Written, no doubt, with a prudent eye on the growth of complaints and litigious threats against doctors, it is nevertheless cast in the moral language of trust and respect. Patients are to be treated as morally autonomous people. Their views are to be listened to and heeded. Their privacy and dignity are to be preserved. Information is to be given to them in ways that they can understand. Their rights to refuse treatment and to become involved in decisions about it are to be respected. Perhaps with the then recent case of Harry Elphick (see Chapter 2) in mind, the guidance emphasizes that doctors are not to allow their views about a patient's lifestyle or worth to prejudice the treatment they offer.

A pan-professional code?

The traditional and relatively straightforward ethical imperatives of autonomy, beneficence and non-maleficence have in recent times been overlaid with at least two complicating innovations. One, which has developed from the increasingly complex interdependence of different professional groups in the health care industry, is the perceived lack of a common ethical foundation uniting all those responsible for the care of patients. Although it has commonly been the medical profession which has subscribed to ethical codes of one kind or another, the inter-connections of modern medical care are now seen by many to be nullifying the usefulness of single-professional codes, particularly in matters to do with the rationing of care. Most medical care was, until recently, a relatively simple matter between doctor and patient, closeted together and largely impervious to events in the world beyond the confines of their mutual society. Increasingly, as the 'stories' in Chapter 6 amply attest, it is no longer like that: many of the most intractable moral difficulties in medicine today arise in the context of complex organizations in which members of multi-disciplinary health care teams are bound by different codes of conduct or none at all (Hurwitz and Richardson, 1997).

Suppose, for example, that an NHS health authority or hospital trust board, working wholly within its legal responsibilities, decided to prohibit or limit the use of an expensive drug. Would it then be ethical for a doctor employed by that hospital to attempt to prescribe the drug for a patient for whom he believed it to offer the best chance of improvement? How, in such a situation, should the ethics of management interact with those of medicine to ensure that the best is done for the particular patient *and also* for all the other patients who might be treated by the trust? Legal issues may also intrude: what, for example, is the nature of a GP's duty to prescribe expensive medicines when the cost of doing so exceeds the cash limits of the primary care group within whose budget she is located (Newdick, 1998)?

Just as importantly, how can the responsibilities that doctors have always assumed for their patients' well-being be safeguarded in health care contexts that are coming increasingly to be dominated by evidence-based medicine and all that this implies (Klein and Maynard, 1998)? The 1997 White Paper proposed the creation of, among many other things, national service frameworks within which local services must develop, a National Institute for Clinical Excellence (NICE) to give a strong lead on effective and efficient treatments, and a Commission for Health Improvement (CHIMP) to oversee the quality of clinical care in local hospitals and health centres (Department of Health, 1997a). To what extent, and why, will doctors be obliged to follow the prescriptions and guidelines of NICE and CHIMP in clinical situations in which they do not believe them to be in their patients' best interests?

Developments such as these are leading to calls for an updating of the traditional ethical codes in the shape of a 'pan-professional oath' to which all those involved in the health care industry can subscribe and which will offer a unified moral framework within which all can practise their skills and arts (Hurwitz and Richardson, 1997). Ethical guidelines that pit one profession against another merely serve to deepen professional divisions, intensify turf wars, and hamper collaborative initiatives. What is needed, some believe, is a code that can cut across disciplinary, professional, organizational and political boundaries and bind together doctors, nurses, other clinicians, managers and executives in their common quest for an ethically justifiable way of using the resources that they severally and corporately control (Berwick *et al.*, 1997).

> The hope is that a single oath for all health care professions could heal split loyalties and ameliorate existing moral tensions . . . Agreeing on such an oath would provide an inclusive opportunity for healthcare workers from different walks of life to speak with one voice for the benefit of patients. (Hurwitz and Richardson, *op. cit.*, p. 1673)

The primary care groups proposed in the 1997 White Paper for England (and their equivalents in Wales and Scotland) furnish an obvious multidisciplinary forum for beginning to develop an ethical consensus of this kind (Marks and Hunter, 1998).

Codes and rationing

A second innovation complicating the traditional rules of moral conduct for doctors is, of course, the part that they and other clinicians are increasingly required to play in the rationing of resources. While traditional ethical codes forestall the exploitation of patients in their clinical encounters with their doctors, they have little to say about a doctor's obligation to share her time justly among all her patients or to have any ethical regard for the social context in which she works (Gillon, 1994). The closest that the Hippocratic Oath comes to any wider considerations of this kind is the blanket requirement to abstain from 'whatever is deleterious and mischievous'. Yet as the 'stories' narrated in Chapter 6 attest, ethical dilemmas arising from a shortage of resources are part and parcel of the everyday experience of clinicians in the NHS. Is it right to withdraw the funding from a patient's course of treatment after it has started simply because the patient joins a fund-holding practice which no longer offers that particular treatment? Is it right for GPs to steer some patients towards a private out-patient consultation in order to conserve the practice budget and to humour important consultants? Is it right for health visitors caring for children with special needs to spend more time with competent families where they are likely to achieve good results than with failing families upon whom much time and other resources could be lavished with little to show? Is it right for a consultant to fail to mention a particular treatment to a patient if he is unsure whether it could be funded? 'We gain little more than self-satisfaction', write Berwick *et al.* 'from codes of conduct that ignore inescapable circumstances such as the social need to place limits on healthcare expenditure, the requirement for management in complex systems, and the strong cultural bias in some nations towards free market solutions' (*op. cit.*, p. 1634).

Revisions to traditional codes have been proposed which do take cognizance of these new realities. Some make their point through parody. 'I will exercise my art not solely for the cure of my patients but I will also take into account the return-on-investment and the cost-benefit ratio . . . since in the overall picture, society will benefit even though an individual patient may suffer some hardship or relapse' (Franzblau and King, quoted in Hurwitz and Richardson, 1997). Others, such as the British Medical Association (BMA) in its draft revision of the Hippocratic Oath, are more serious in their language. 'I will use my training and professional standing to improve the community in which I work. I will treat patients equitably and support a fair and humane distribution of health resources . . . I will strive to change laws which are contrary to patients' interests . . .' (British Medical Association, 1997, p. 26). In issuing its draft revision, the BMA committed itself to pressing for its adoption on a worldwide basis.

The limitation in all such ethical codes, however, lies in their inability to provide answers to specific ethical problems (Limentani, 1998). They can certainly give a necessary shape and structure to the moral environment in which health care is set, but they can never be so tightly drawn as to remove the need for the exercise of ethical choice by individual doctors, nurses, physiotherapists, and others. The wording of the BMA's draft revision of the Hippocratic Oath may appear impressively reassuring, but what would it mean for a doctor to 'treat patients equitably' or to 'support a fair distribution of health resources'? Who is to say whether or not a given budgetary allocation, determined by a legally constituted health authority, is 'contrary to the interests of patients'? How would the BMA's revision have helped the paediatricians treating Jaymee Bowen, who had to weigh the cost of an innovative treatment against its low (but not zero) probability of success and the pain it might cause? How would it have helped the renal physicians who were responsible for the unpromising patient in Oxford to determine the point at which to discontinue his dialysis (see Chapter 2)?

What appears to be involved in such difficult matters is a conflict between moral concerns that operate at different levels (Gillon, 1994). Clinicians have a primary moral obligation to treat the individual patients before them. Managers have a primary moral obligation to see that public resources are not wasted. Politicians have a primary moral obligation to use the nation's resources fairly and to balance the reasonable interests and expectations of different sections of society. It is as if, to use Calabresi and Bobbitt's (1978) metaphor, a juggler is trying to keep more balls in the air than is humanly possible. A sensible way forward, Gillon argues, is to abandon the fruitless search for the grand solution until we are much more skilled in the ethical arts, and to concentrate instead on finding pragmatic ways of reconciling the competing moral concerns in all the arenas, large and small, in which they surface.

This may require us, first, to recognize the immense complexity of the problem and to resist the temptation to resort to simple solutions. Next, it may mean accepting that, until the skills of the metaphorical juggler have improved, some balls will inevitably fall to the ground from time to time. The honest pursuit of justice will always leave some people dissatisfied. It is regrettable whenever it occurs, and all reasonable actions should be taken to minimize its adverse consequences; but it cannot be helped. And finally it requires us to find ways of developing the juggler's capacity to cope with an ever increasing number of balls. These may include, as we noted above, the search for reformulations of traditional moral codes that take realistic account of the corporate context of modern medicine and the development of what Hurwitz and Richardson (1997) have called pan-professional oaths.

5

Ethics and the outcomes of health care rationing

Classifying the outcomes of care

The importance of outcomes

The arguments in the two preceding chapters have drawn attention to some of the moral questions about rationing that seem to arise from the ways in which health care services are structured and operated. Are their structures likely to produce a fair distribution of scarce resources, and are their decision-making processes ethically defensible? There is, however, a third way of looking at health services which may also raise moral questions about rationing, and that is in terms of the results or the effects which they produce. In Donabedian's (1980) language they are the outcomes of care. Health services may, in principle, be striving to achieve a variety of different outcomes, from the saving of individual life to the optimization of the health of the community as a whole. In an ideal world all of these objectives would be pursued. In the real world of resource constraints, however, the ideal is just that – an ideal. Choices must sometimes be made, if only by default, between a number of different possible outcomes, raising the question of whether some objectives are morally to be preferred to others in situations where, realistically, they cannot all be achieved.

To focus the morality of rationing on the outcomes of care is, arguably, to address the issues at their most profound level, for we may feel that what ultimately count are neither the structures of care nor their processes but the effects they produce on the everyday lives and experiences of people. Health services are to be admired and approved neither for their anatomy nor for their physiology but for the beneficial impact they achieve on people's health. The difficulty, however, lies in the greater ease with which we can usually understand structures and processes than outcomes. Outcomes are elusive things. Even at the level of individual patients, the valid attribution of an improvement in health to the effects of an antecedent treatment may sometimes be tricky, and at a population level, where ethical questions are most likely to be located, the difficulties multiply. It is commonplace to observe that, among populations as a whole, measurable improvements in health are likely to reflect a variety of social, economic, environmental, educational and occupational changes, among which the care provided by the NHS is only one (and in some cases not even the major) determinant.

Notwithstanding the delicacy that may be required to tickle this particular trout, some of the most troublesome arguments in the morality of health care rationing require us to do just that. Since they hinge in part around the question of whether one type of outcome is morally to be preferred to another in situations where they may come into conflict, we must first describe the different ways in which the outcomes of care can be understood. Three are usually singled out for special scrutiny in this particular corner of the moral maze: outcome as meeting individual needs, outcome as maximizing the health gain, and outcome as narrowing the health gap.

Outcome as meeting individual needs

First, we can think about the effects of health care in terms of meeting the health needs of *individuals*. Doctors and other clinicians work mainly with individual people. They are in the business of making them better when they are ill and of helping them to remain well thereafter. To be sure, the objective is not always achieved. Patients may fail to improve for all sorts of reasons unconnected with the quality of the care they receive. But however successful or otherwise the treatment may be, the central objective is usually quite clear: to improve the health of the individual patient by addressing the needs that he or she presents. The goal of care is defined, and its effectiveness is measured, by the impact it has upon the well-being of individual patients.

Within this core task of medical practice, however, other views about the purposes and objectives of health care can be discerned which move the focus of outcome away from individual patients to groups or populations of patients. The broad objective remains of meeting the variety of needs that patients present, but shifts occur in policy prescriptions of what should be done, to whom, and in what order. Two examples of the shift in focus from the individual to the group, which are of particular importance in the context of rationing because of their centrality to the policy objectives of the 1997 Labour government, can be described as 'maximizing the health gain' and 'narrowing the health gap'.

Outcome as maximizing the health gain

The origins of the notion of 'health gain' are difficult to fix with much precision. They are located partly in traditional epidemiological concerns with the levels and changes of health among populations (Morris, 1975), partly in the stream of economic analysis that strives to relate the costs of care to the effects which it achieves (Culyer, 1976), and partly in the early attempts to bring these epidemiological and economic streams together in public health policy (Lalonde, 1975). The introduction of the so-called internal market in the NHS in the early 1990s, based as it was on a network of contracts between the separated purchasers and providers of care, gave substance to the idea of health gain by requiring purchasers to measure the health changes accruing from the money they were spending (NHS Management Executive, 1990). By 1998 it had become an explicit aim of government policy 'to improve the health of the population *as a whole* by increasing the length of people's lives and the number of years people spend free from illness' (Department of Health, 1998, p. 5, emphasis added).

Yet to focus in this way upon the health of people *en masse* may be to undercut the traditional concerns of medical practice in meeting the needs of *individual* patients. Individual lives may be accorded a lesser value than statistical lives. A simple illustration will make the point – though the realities, of course, are infinitely more complex. Imagine a group of ten patients suffering from a particular condition. Imagine further that the budget available for their treatment is £1,000. Of the group of ten patients, two are in an advanced stage of the disease. Their lives could both be extended by five years, but as the cost of treating them would be £500 each, to do so would consume the entire budget. The remaining eight patients are in an earlier stage of the disease. Their lives could all be extended by ten years, but as the cost of treating them would be £125 each, to do so would also consume the entire budget. No other relevant differences exist between the two sub-groups of patients.

What should the health service be trying to achieve in such a situation? The formal aim of the government to 'improve the health of the population as a whole by increasing the length of people's lives' would best be achieved by treating the eight patients with the more promising prognoses and leaving the other two to die. By doing so, a further 80 years of life could be gained for the £1,000 that is available for their treatment. Were the money to be spent in any other way, fewer extra years of life would be gained. Yet what about the two patients whose individual needs would be brushed aside in the pursuit of the greatest aggregate outcome? They are, in one sense, in greater medical need than the majority, for in them the disease is more advanced. Their lives are under threat. Are their greater needs to be sacrificed in order to, as the White Paper put it, 'improve the health of the population [group] as a whole'? How could such a choice be reconciled with the seemingly widespread view, discussed in Chapter 2, that far from penalizing them, the intensity of people's needs for care is a legitimate basis for discriminating *in their favour*? Does it matter what the two patients themselves might feel about being used as pawns in a wider social policy? Does it matter what their doctors might feel about it? There are, it seems, important ethical problems lurking beneath the apparently uncontentious aim of maximizing the health gain of the population *as a whole*.

Outcome as narrowing the health gap

Similar concerns may arise with the parallel objective of 'narrowing the health gap'. It has long been known that illness, disability and premature death do not occur evenly among the population (Townsend and Davidson, 1982). Almost however 'social class' is defined, those who find themselves at the lower end of the spectrum of social advantage suffer worse health and are more likely to die at younger ages than those in the upper reaches; and the NHS, far from reducing such differences, has in many respects failed even to prevent them from widening (Drever and Whitehead, 1997). For much of the 1980s and 1990s the 'health gap' (as the phenomenon came to be known) was either denied or deemed to be beyond the effective scope of public policy. What health care activists wanted to call 'health inequalities' was transmuted into the ideologically more neutral notion of 'health differences' which were portrayed as resulting in part from the ways that people voluntarily chose to lead their lives. The Labour government of 1997 promised a different and more pro-active approach to the gap, formally committing itself in 1998 to 'improve the health of the worst off in society and to narrow the health gap' (Department of Health, 1998, p. 5).

Yet as with the related objective of improving the health of the population as a whole, policies that seek to change the social distribution of illness and early death may, by focusing on population-based measures of outcome, collide with ideas about justice for individuals. Imagine another group of ten patients suffering from the same condition at the same stage of development. Five are located at the upper end of the spectrum of social advantage (however it is defined) and five at the lower end. The appropriate treatment costs £200 for each patient, and a budget of £1,000 is available for the group. The policy objective of 'narrowing the health gap' would require more of the budget to be spent on the five socially disadvantaged patients than on the others. This might be done by using the whole of the budget for their treatment; or, less radically, it might be done by treating four or three of them and only one or two of the socially more advantaged patients. All else being equal, the effect would be a modest contribution towards a narrowing of the health gap.

Yet what, in this imagined scenario, are we to make of the fate of the more advantaged patients, all (or some) of whom would be denied the treatment they needed as individuals in order to achieve a collective outcome? Would it be ethically acceptable to discriminate against these patients *solely* because of their social or economic position in society? Do they not also have rights in a health service that has traditionally proclaimed a person's social class to be irrelevant to his chances of gaining access to the care he needs? If it is morally unacceptable to discriminate against socially less advantaged patients *simply* because of their lesser advantage, is it not equally unacceptable to discriminate against socially more advantaged patients *simply* because of their greater advantage?

These three ways of looking at the outcomes of health care (meeting individual patients' needs, maximizing the health gain and narrowing the health gap) relate to the rationing of health care in different ways and they appear to give rise to tricky moral questions. It seems intuitively right that, all else being equal, scarce resources (whether in health care or any other area of human activity) should be used in ways that will produce the most good. The devil lies in the detail of adjudicating between different notions of what is 'good'.

Meeting the health care needs of individuals

Needs and resources

Basic though it is to the purposes of a health care system, meeting the health care needs of individuals is far from being a straightforward and uncomplicated objective. 'Need' is an infuriating word: we cannot, it seems, manage without it yet we seem to have great difficulty in defining it in ways that make it useful in public debate. To begin with, it appears to be relatively straightforward. If I suffer severe abdominal pain and a doctor diagnoses appendicitis, then I may fairly claim to need an operation to remove the troublesome organ. My claim rests upon two considerations: that without the operation my condition is expected to get very much worse but that with the operation I could expect to make a full recovery. So far so good; but suppose that my appendix starts to trouble me in a remote area far removed from *any* surgeon, much less a competent one working in a fully equipped theatre. I may be on a walking holiday in the Himalayan foothills or helping in a refugee camp in a remote part of Africa or sailing in a round-the-world yacht race. Do I still need an operation, even though, for all practical purposes, my chances of getting it within a reasonable period of time are zero?

One answer, plainly, is yes: I do still need the operation, but it is a need that cannot be met in the particular circumstance in which I happen to find myself. The fact that it cannot be met does not detract from my intrinsic state of need, and if my health suffers because of my inability to reach a surgeon, then it becomes a case of unmet need, possibly with a tragic outcome. But that is not the only answer, for if a surgeon were unavailable, then my definition of what I needed would shift. Rather than having an unmet need for surgical treatment, I would have an active need for an alternative form of care that *might* be available. Although surgery is normally the treatment of choice in appendicitis, it is not the only one: medical treatment by antibiotics and the drainage of gastric juices may be effective in certain cases, at least until surgery can be carried out, and I would certainly find it preferable to twiddling my thumbs. The physician in the group with which I am travelling, and who made the diagnosis of appendicitis, will probably have the antibiotics and may possibly have the drainage equipment.

If, however, even that is unavailable and my condition begins to look quite serious, my need may change again. If the likely outcome is that I will die of peritonitis if nothing at all is done, then *any* kind of intervention by the doctor in the group, however desperate it may be by normal clinical standards, may be better than nothing. By now my need is very basic, but no less real for that. When a female passenger collapsed with a punctured lung on a scheduled air flight from Hong Kong to London and her condition destabilized quite quickly, she found herself needing not the pristine facilities of a modern operating suite but precisely what happened to be available on the aircraft at the time: a consultant surgeon and various pieces of makeshift equipment sterilized with brandy from the drinks trolley. Her primary need for modern surgical intervention remained, but it was, for all practical purposes, overtaken by a qualitatively different kind of need dictated by her faltering condition in unusual circumstances. What in more ordinary circumstances would never have been seen as the care she needed became, in the transformed conditions in which she found herself, a very pressing need indeed.

The needs that people have for care are not, then, immutable. They may change as circumstances change. In particular, they may change in response to the shifting availability of the resources required to meet them. The example is given in the district nurse's 'story' in Chapter 6 of an elderly lady with poor bladder control whose arthritis prevents a speedy access to the toilet. There is a local policy of supplying incontinence pads free of charge, but only to patients with very debilitating illnesses or whose continence problems are a complication of surgery. She does not fall into either category, but neither can she afford to pay privately for a regular supply of the pads. In any case, she would be unable to get out to buy them. As a result, she is often wet and suffers from extensive skin sores. What is her need in such a situation? Her most obvious need is for the care of her sores by a district nurse. But she may also be said to have a different kind of need that is just as authentic: the need for a free supply of incontinence pads, or, if the health authority persists in adhering rigidly to its exclusion categories, the need for the financial resources and the transport that would allow her to buy them privately. That neither pads nor money are likely to materialize in no way lessens her need for them.

Needs and the health care system

Yet another facet of the notion of need is revealed by those whose health care needs span a number of different services. A healthy young man with no history of major illness is made redundant from his job. Even after a long period of time, he is unable to find work. His finances begin to wobble and his house is repossessed by the building society. His family has to split up for the time being, his wife and children going to live with her parents while he searches for work. He finds himself becoming lethargic and depressed. He see less and less of his wife and children and feels more and more stressed. His blood pressure rises and he begins to entertain suicidal thoughts. His wife, too, develops an almost continual stream of minor complaints and his children are showing signs of behavioural disturbance.

The health service is committed to 'meeting the needs' of this patient and his family; but what are they? Most obviously, they need to have their physical and mental symptoms investigated and treated in appropriate ways. But to do no more than that would be to leave untouched the well-springs of their problems. The man has a deeper set of needs which, if not addressed, may cause his health problems to reappear and further costs to be incurred in their treatment. He needs a job. He needs to find a way of being able to live with his family again. He may need help in rebuilding his relationship with his wife. He needs to have hope that suitable housing will be found which is within his budget. Such needs are no less real for being difficult to quantify, and unless they are met, his own health and that of his family may be at further risk.

But are they needs that should be met through the health care system? They are certainly needs that may affect the man's current and future prospects of good health; but does it follow that they should therefore be met from the resources of the NHS? Intuitively, it seems reasonable that the NHS should provide whatever help the man may need in rebuilding his relationships with his family, for 'counselling' services are not too far removed from psychiatric care, and in any case such services are now available in many general practices. To expect the NHS to help resolve his needs for work and accommodation may, however, strike us as an expectation too far. We can certainly appreciate the deleterious impact that his lack of work and accommodation is having on his own health and that of his family, but we may feel that the responsibility for doing something about them lies elsewhere.

To say that, however, is to set limits to the responsibility of the health care system for meeting people's health care needs. Bad housing, for example, is a significant cause of widespread and varied ill health (Best, 1995), but the responsibility of the NHS is limited to dealing with the consequences rather than removing the causes. Yet the same is not the case with, say, dietary deficiencies of one sort or another. These, too, are major causes of serious morbidity and early death; but here the NHS does accept a responsibility for trying to change the way that people eat. Weight-control clinics are often provided in general practices, healthy eating campaigns are mounted by the Department of Health, and patients who are too heavy or too light are counselled about their eating as part of their personal medical care. Where, then, are the limits drawn? If the core task of the service is to 'meet individual people's health care needs', including their need to prevent ill health in the future, where lies the point beyond which the service can legitimately decline to offer help? Which of their various health care needs should patients *not* expect the NHS to meet?

The elasticity of need

The ostensibly straightforward notion with which we began this discussion, that the NHS is there to 'fix people's needs', is, on reflection, more complicated than it seems at first glance. At one level it *is* straightforward: we 'need' the care that will be effective in improving our current state of health and protecting our future state. We need whatever it may take to ensure an acceptable level of 'flourishing'; and it is the job of the health care system and those who work in it to provide it. Yet need is an elastic notion, expanding and contracting in response to what is possible, what is affordable, and what is available. It is not like a lump of plasticine, of uniform texture and consistency. It is not capable of being cut into pieces, the volumes or weights of which can be measured precisely in relation to all the others. To argue, then, that health care should be rationed in proportion to people's needs is to open a particularly problematic can of worms, some of which carry the label 'conceptual' and others the label 'methodological'.

It was suggested in Chapter 2, for example, that the relative intensity of the needs of different patients is widely seen as a morally acceptable basis for choosing between them in situations where choices must (albeit regrettably) be made. To recall the illustration used in that chapter, it seems 'obviously right' that a GP should spend much more of his time attending a young woman with breast cancer than an old man with a sore throat. But to have chosen such a sharp contrast was deliberately to simplify a choice that all too often is far from simple in reality. How are we to compare situations of need that are intrinsically incommensurable? How are we to adjudicate between the need of an elderly arthritic lady for a free supply of incontinence pads and that of a young man for symptomatic treatment of AIDS? How can the prevention of future ill health in a family which is breaking apart be balanced against that of a stable family coping with a child with special needs? How can patients whose health care needs fall unambiguously within the purview of the NHS be compared with those whose health would benefit more than anything from better housing, a cleaner environment or a minimum wage?

Nor does the business of rationing health care on the basis of people's needs become any easier by switching our focus away from the choices that may have to be made between individuals to the design of systems of care that meet particular criteria of justice. One such system, proposed by Doyal (1995), was examined in Chapter 3. At the heart of Doyal's notion of a morally justifiable structure of health care is the idea that if cuts have to be made or resources rationed it should be done evenly across all categories of clinical need. Services for people with mental health needs, for example, should be cut proportionally no more, or no less, than those for patients needing, say, open heart surgery. Doyal illustrates the point through such discrete and quantifiable segments of need as 'heart disease, kidney disease, orthopaedic problems, psychiatric illness, and so on' (*op. cit.*, p. 276). Each, he argues, should be cut in bad times and expanded in good times by a statistically comparable proportion.

For a health authority to do this, however, is to assume the feasibility of precisely what we have argued cannot easily be done – slicing up a fixed mass of 'need for health care' into discrete and quantifiable segments of uniform texture and consistency. How, for example, would the need of the elderly incontinent lady or the disintegrating family be dealt with in such a schema? How could the services used by a family with a severely handicapped child be cut by the same proportion as those involved in the treatment of a failed suicide? Some needs *may* be capable of compartmentalizing in this way – for various elective surgical procedures, for sub-fertility treatment, for renal dialysis, and so on. But as the 'stories' in Chapter 6 reveal, many needs are far too complex, fluid and overlapping with each other to turn Doyal's principle into a workable guideline across the whole range of what the NHS offers. We seem to be in precisely the position described at the opening of this section: we find it difficult to talk about the ethics of health care without invoking the idea of need, but we find it even more difficult to handle it in ways that relate to the realities of care in the NHS.

Maximizing the health gain

Health gain, resources and rationing

At the heart of the notion of 'health gain' is the idea that health care services should be provided and managed in ways that will maximize the health of those who use them. Put in this way, the idea seems unexceptionable. The whole point of having a health service is to keep people healthy in the first place, restore them to good health when they become ill, and care for their symptoms when cures are lacking. That is also, broadly, the rationale of the clinical professions: as Sacket has put it, 'doctors . . . identify and apply the most efficacious interventions to maximise the quality and quantity of life for individual patients . . .' (Sacket *et al.*, 1996, p. 72). There is, however, a nasty sting in the tail of Sacket's formulation of the doctor's task: 'this may raise rather than lower the cost of their care' (*op. cit.*, p. 72). In an ideal world, where resources flowed freely and rationing was an unspeakable monster confined to the safety of fairy tales, health care services could strive to maximize the quantity and quality of each patient's life whatever the cost. Clinical decisions could be taken solely on the basis of their impact on the health of patients. Resource constraints would not enter into the picture. Yet because the real world is one in which resources *are* constrained and doctors *are* obliged to take account of the costs of their work, the notion of 'health gain' must be modified: not simply to maximize the health of those who use the health service, but to maximize health within whatever pot of resources is available. To do so is inevitably to shift the focus away from individual patients towards groups or populations of patients; and the altered focus may yield a very different image.

Maynard (1997) offers a schematic example. Suppose there are two alternative therapies, A and B, which, on the basis of the best available evidence, are likely to produce increased life expectancies of five and ten years respectively. Suppose further that neither treatment offers a better quality of life than the other. If costs are ignored and the choice of treatment is based *only* on the maximization of the expected quantity and quality of life, then treatment B will be selected. It will be the treatment of choice, consistent with the requirements of evidence-based medicine. But suppose, next, that therapy A costs £1,500 and therapy B £7,000. By choosing A, a doctor will be able to secure one extra year of 'good' quality life for £300, while the choice of B will secure the same outcome for £700. To put it the other way round, from a budget of, say, £100,000 for the treatment of this particular condition, therapy A will yield an expected 333 extra years of life while B will yield only 143 extra years. The conclusion, then, is quite dramatic: by ignoring cost, therapy B is twice as good as A; but *within the available level of resource*, A appears to be more than twice as good as B.

Utilitarianism

All of this is, at root, to locate the debate about health care rationing within the lengthy tradition of utilitarianism, a prominent strand in English philosophical thought that flourished between the mid-eighteenth and mid-nineteenth centuries. Though classical utilitarianism is more a collection of related ideas than a cohesive and unitary system, its broad themes can be summarized with sufficient clarity for the present purpose. Plamenatz (1966) offers four propositions about utilitarianism which, broadly, box the compass for us. The first is that pleasure is good and desirable for its own sake; the second is that the equal pleasures of two or more men are equally good; the third is that any action is right if, under the circumstances, it produces the greatest possible amount of happiness; and the fourth is that the web of reciprocal obligations between citizens and government is independent of the way that government acquires power or maintains it. In populist shorthand, utilitarianism is about the greatest happiness of the greatest number.

Strictly speaking, theories about the arrangement of health care resources in ways that will maximize the quantity and quality of people's lives are neo-utilitarian rather than classically utilitarian. In place of pleasure and happiness they put the length and quality of life. They are, it may be said, concerned with maximizing welfare rather than happiness (and, as will be seen, a great deal hinges on the way that 'welfare' is defined). Nevertheless, the guiding principle is the same: the right and rational course of action in a situation where resources are insufficient to maximize the health of *individuals* is to maximize the health of the population or group *as a whole*.

The Quality Adjusted Life Year (QALY)

Calculating the QALY

This principle has been worked through most rigorously and most famously in the Quality Adjusted Life Year (QALY), a tool that claims to offer a rational, utilitarian method of allocating health care resources in an optimal and morally defensible way. Though potentially complex in its construction and application, the basic elements of the QALY can be readily understood. Purporting to show the relative health benefits that will accrue from different ways of allocating a fixed volume of health care resources, the first step involves the estimation (using whatever clinical or epidemiological data might be to hand) of the additional years of life that can typically be expected to result from a particular medical or surgical procedure.

Standard life-tables of this kind have been calculated and used for many years (Smith, 1987), but the QALY goes a step further by weighting the expected *quantity* of life following the procedure by an indication of its *quality*. There is here, perhaps, an implicit acknowledgement of the utilitarian origins of the tool: what counts for most people is not just being alive but having some degree of pleasure or happiness in their lives. The QALY acknowledges this by building the notion of 'quality of life' into the method. In principle, it could be done in many different ways. In practice, many quality-of-life weightings have built upon the pioneering work of Rosser (Rosser and Watts, 1972; Rosser and Kind, 1978). Noting from her observational work that diverse groups of people – including doctors – tended to define the severity of illness in terms of the disability it caused (through impaired mobility and function) and the distress it inflicted (through anxiety and pain), Rosser developed an index of illness states that combined disability and distress into a scale of health states ranging from 0 to 1.0. Zero denotes death (though it is perfectly possible to imagine states worse than death which would have a negative value); 1.0 denotes the total absence of disability and distress; and the intermediate points denote varying combinations of disability and distress.

Although there are many variations on the initial scale developed by Rosser, the principles of their construction are similar. Once a quality-of-life scale has been worked out and the realism of its assumptions tested on various groups of subjects (Gudex and Kind, 1988), it is multiplied by the expected number of years of life remaining before and after a particular treatment is given or procedure carried out. The difference between the two computations is the QALY score that is attached to the treatment. If, for example, patients typically have two years of life expectancy before undergoing a procedure and the quality of those years is rated as 0.4, the pre-treatment score is 0.8 (i.e. 2 × 0.4). If the expectation of life following treatment increases to ten years and their quality is raised to 0.6, the post-treatment score is 6.0 (10 × 0.6). The QALY value for that procedure is then the difference between the two scores: 5.2 (6.0 − 0.8). If, on the other hand, the treatment is expected to produce only three extra years of life but their quality is rated as 0.8, then the post-treatment score changes to 2.4 (3 × 0.8) and the QALY value for the procedure reduces to 1.6 (2.4 − 0.8). Simple adjustments can obviously be made to the calculations to allow for the possibility that the quality of life may change throughout the expected survival period. It will be apparent from these two examples that crucial to the whole thing is the assumption that the quantity and quality of life are commensurable and can be traded off against each other. In the world of QALYs, nine years of life of quality 0.4 is exactly equivalent to six years of life of quality 0.6.

QALY league tables

The next step in the process is to calculate the average cost of generating one QALY from each particular treatment or procedure. If, for example, treatment S costs £1,000 and has a QALY value of 6.0, then the cost per QALY for that treatment is £167. That is how much it costs to generate one quality adjusted life year through the treatment. If, by contrast, treatment T costs £8,000 and has a QALY value of only 3.0, then the cost per QALY for that treatment is £2,667. The final step, flowing with remorseless logic from the calculation of cost per QALY for different treatments, is to array all the treatments in a league table, ordered in their ascending cost per QALY. For such a table to be valid, all the QALY calculations in it must be strictly comparable: they must, for example, use identical measures of the anticipated quality of life and their costs must relate to comparable treatment settings and be based on the same year (Mason, Drummond and Torrance, 1993). Typical of the many such tables that have been published over the last decade is that compiled by Maynard (1991). The best value for money in this table was offered by treatments such as neurosurgical intervention for head injury (£220 per QALY at 1990 prices), GP advice to stop smoking (£270), pacemaker implantation (£1,100) and bypass graft for severe angina (£2,090). In the middle of the range of cost per QALY were cholesterol testing and treatment of adults aged 25–39 (£14,150), home haemodialysis (£17,260) and bypass graft for moderate angina (£18,830). At the bottom of the table were neurosurgical intervention for malignant tumours (£107,780) and drug treatment for anaemia in patients undergoing dialysis using Erythropoietin (£126,290).

The application of QALYs

So much for the nuts and bolts of QALYs. As modern exponents of the utilitarian tradition, their supporters believe them to have a pivotal (though not decisive) role in the rationing choices that have to be made in the NHS. If resources are tight, and if the government is committed to a policy of maximizing the health of the population as a whole, then QALYs are seen to offer as rational a basis as any other for guiding the difficult choices that have to be made. While they could, in principle, be used for both first-order and second-order rationing decisions, their value is more likely to be felt at the higher level. QALYs are good at indicating whether more resources should be invested in, say, haemodialysis than in hip replacements. They are less good at showing whether Mrs G, who needs dialysis, should be given greater priority in treatment than Mrs H, who needs a new hip. This is partly because QALYs necessarily deal in statistical averages rather than individual lives, but mainly because the choices that may have to be made between haemodialysis and hip replacements are always likely to be choices between *services* rather than between *patients*. It is much easier to imagine the circumstances in which a health authority may be faced with an investment decision between one service or the other than it is to think of a real-life situation in which a clinical team might be required to make a similar choice between one patient and another. If QALYs have value, it lies in the light they can shed upon the allocation of resources among competing treatment programmes.

There is an aura of logic, and even of moral rectitude, about QALYs that is strongly persuasive. Who could reasonably deny the proposition that scarce resources should be used where they can do the most good? The problem, of course, lies in the conflict of views about what constitutes 'the most good'; and it is here that the qualms about QALYs begin to surface. The critiques fall, broadly, into two groups: methodological and ethical.

Methodological critiques

From a methodological standpoint, QALYs have been criticized as being less rational and more subjective than their supporters imply (Loomes and McKenzie, 1989). Even if QALYs are justified in whatever it is they are trying to measure, the validity and the reliability of their measurements can be questioned (Ashmore, Mulkay and Pinch, 1989). How can such an immensely complex, subjective and multi-faceted concept as 'quality of life' possibly be reduced to a single numerical value between 0 and 1.0 – and done, moreover, in a way that can fairly be applied to all patients undergoing each defined treatment? How accurate, and how meaningful, are the estimates about the average survival times and the expected quality of life following each treatment? How sensitive are the average computed costs of the different treatments, and how can we be sure that the costs of all the treatments in any particular league table have been defined and calculated in precisely the same way and relate to precisely the same dates? How, in any case, can QALY league tables keep pace with rapid changes in the costs and the outcomes of clinical practice without the investment of huge sums of research money? Without satisfactory answers to such questions, the use of QALYs must raise precisely the same kind of ethical doubt that would be raised by *any* procedure which has been inadequately tested.

A related matter of methodological concern to the critics of QALYs is the very basis on which they are constructed. The criterion of 'quality of life', upon which so much of the credibility of the QALY rests, is composed of two elements: disability and distress. The weights that are attached to them derive from the values of the small and selective groups of people who are involved in the development of the index. Such values, however, may differ from those held by other, more representative groups of people, particularly those who are most likely to be affected by the application of QALYs to the rationing of care. As Nord (1992) points out, for example, a life in a wheelchair is considered by the QALY not only to be less healthy than a life without disability, but also of less value. Accordingly, patients who are likely to be alive but disabled following treatment will suffer discrimination in a QALY calculation – a position that is both ethically contestable and repugnant to disabled people themselves (Harris, 1987).

Such considerations may lead in a number of directions. In the US, the federal government has flatly rejected all attempts to ration publicly funded health care programmes incorporating quality-of-life indicators because of their probable violation of the rights of disabled people (Honigsbaum, Holmström and Calltorp, 1997, p. 9). Others, by contrast, have sought to retain the utilitarian basis of the QALY while purging it of its discriminatory overtones. One example is the disability adjusted life year (the DALY), incorporating the judgments that disabled people themselves make about the quality of their own lives (rather than the judgments which able-bodied people make on their behalf). Another example is the saved young life equivalent (SAVE), reflecting not only the aggregate amount of health gained by people undergoing particular treatments but also the social value that representative citizens would place upon the gains, using as the baseline the 'absolute value' that is presumed to be accorded to the saving of life and the restoration of full health in a young person (Nord, 1992).

Moral critiques

It is, however, the utilitarian basis of the QALY and its derivatives that has brought it under attack from moral as well as from methodological quarters. At the heart of the moral concern over QALYs is the fact that, since they measure people's capacity to benefit from care rather than their need for it, they have little to say about the *justice* of any particular way of distributing health care (Lockwood, 1988). Justice, we may feel, requires us at least to try to provide services in proportion to people's need for them; utilitarianism, by contrast, requires services to be provided in proportion to people's ability to benefit from them. When purely utilitarian considerations are allowed to dominate, the results can be, quite simply, wrong. A stylized example will illustrate the point. Imagine that two young men are on the point of death because of a shortage of donor organs. One needs a new heart and the other a new liver. In each case a transplant operation is judged to be suitable, with the expectation of good results. At this point, a third young man is admitted to the accident and emergency department of the hospital in which the other two are patients. He has multiple head injuries sustained in a motor-cycle accident and he is carrying an organ donor card. The assessment of his condition is bleak: he needs immediate surgical intervention to stabilize his condition, and his extensive brain damage is giving rise to serious concern about the quality of his life were he to survive. If he were allowed to die, his heart and liver would be available for transplantation into the other two patients; but if he were given emergency surgery in an attempt to save his own life, the others may die first.

If, in this imagined situation, the greatest possible extension of human life is judged to be a supreme value in society, then 'society' would be justified in maximizing this value by allowing the third man to die and using his organs to 'save' the lives of the other two. It would be the utilitarian solution because the total expected benefit from treating the two would exceed the total expected benefit from treating the one. It would achieve the maximum quantity, and possibly also quality, of life preserved – and it might do so, moreover, at least cost. Yet were this to happen, we would rightly feel a sense of moral outrage, for the third man also has a proper claim on the community's resources which cannot simply be pushed aside in the name of a greater good. Having been admitted to the hospital in a life-threatening state of need, the hospital is morally bound to do whatever it reasonably can to meet his dire individual need. It is entirely irrelevant to the hospital's obligation towards him that his organs may be instrumental in extending the lives of two other patients. The possibility of transplantation becomes a consideration only if, after all the appropriate care has been given, a patient dies. It can never be ethical to allow the promise of a cull of organs to influence the way a patient is treated, and it is plainly wrong for doctors to take any positive steps to hasten the deaths of patients whose organs may be suitable for transplantation. By the same token, it must be equally wrong for them to withhold treatment in the hope or expectation of the availability of viable organs.

To fail to give due weight to the argument from justice is to allow 'need' to be overridden by 'benefit'. Whenever health care resources are allocated in ways that are likely to produce the best aggregate outcome, then services which generally produce a good outcome are always likely to be given priority over services producing lesser benefits. Often, however, these are precisely the services required by patients in the greatest need. Under a utilitarian approach, the principle of 'giving to each according to his need' is supplanted by the alternative principle of 'giving to each according to his capacity to benefit'.

The QALY and the ethics of outcomes

It is here that the QALY comes under the ethical microscope, for it is not directly sensitive to people's needs. If Mrs G has end-stage renal disease and a donor kidney is not available, her need for haemodialysis is of the highest order, for without it she will die and there is no greater threat to human flourishing than the imminence of death. If Mrs H, by contrast, has an arthritic hip, she may be in considerable pain and her movement may be severely restricted; but her need for treatment, though of course real, would scarcely be seen as matching that of Mrs G. Yet under every QALY calculation, hip replacements have been shown consistently to offer much better value for money than either home or hospital dialysis; and if the health authority in which both Mrs G and Mrs H reside has followed the utilitarian guidelines and invested more heavily in hip replacements than in dialysis facilities, then Mrs G's claims on the resources of the NHS (and the claims of all other such patients of whom she is the exemplar) will be systematically devalued in comparison to those of the relatively less needy Mrs H (and all those of whom *she* is the exemplar).

None of this is to say that the utilitarian approach to rationing is intrinsically wrong or even that it is always less desirable than one which attempts to adjudicate between people's needs. It does, however, indicate that the two must be kept apart and that each must be consciously evaluated in relation to the other as guiding principles in the rationing of health care resources. Obvious though this may seem, the distinction between need and the capacity to benefit can all too easily be elided. A research paper written by health economists and published by the National Association of Health Authorities and Trusts in 1992 actually went so far as to say that 'a more sophisticated approach to needs assessment involves *equating* need with ability to benefit . . . indeed, there is a clear advantage to this approach over that which equates need with illness' (Mooney *et al.*, 1992, p. 10, emphasis added). Such a view is bad news for those who are seriously ill, particularly those whose illnesses, even after treatment, are likely to leave them with a poor prognosis. To equate 'need' with 'ability to benefit' is to offer a justification for the utilitarianism of QALYs on misleading grounds, for 'ability to benefit' has no intrinsic or systematic relationship to need. There may well be instances (appendicitis being an obvious example) in which the intensity of the need and the expected response to treatment will both be high. In other cases, however, as a perusal of any of the published QALY league tables suggests, the greater a patient's need, the less rosy may be the outcome of care, particularly when treatment is started at a later stage in the disease process (New and Le Grand, 1996, p. 58).

Narrowing the health gap

Justice and distribution of health care resources

Just as the policy aim of maximizing the health of the population appears, intuitively, to be a good thing, so too does the parallel aim of narrowing the health gap. That high rates of illness and early death are disproportionately concentrated among families living in sub-standard housing or with low incomes or with poor job prospects offends our sense of fairness. That such inequalities have actually widened in many respects throughout the 50 years of the NHS may strike us as an even greater cause for social concern, justifying government action to halt and reverse the trend. Yet just as the goal of the maximization of health outcomes gives rise to important moral concerns, so too does that of the minimization of health inequalities; for it too, by placing a high value on population-based measures of outcome, may fail to give due attention to what we may see as one of the fundamental requirements of justice, namely that patients should be treated equally in relation to their needs, whatever their social or economic status.

There are, of course, obvious circumstances under which justice is not only heeded but even advanced by sharing out the resources for health care in ways that are intended to reduce the health gap. Relative to national averages, some parts of the United Kingdom have experienced persistently high levels of illness and premature death, together with low levels of spending on health care. That this is unfair has been explicitly acknowledged since the mid-1970s, when policies were begun to rearrange the financial resources of the NHS in ways designed, over time, to give each regional and area health authority a fairer allocation in relation to its needs (Department of Health and Social Security, 1976b). At the regional level, at least, these policies have succeeded in bringing the health regions closer to the target share of the national cake that each *would* receive *if* the cake were divided in strict proportion to its need (measured mainly, though not entirely, through age-adjusted death rates). Regions receiving more than their 'fair' share have moved downwards towards their targets, while those receiving less have moved upwards (Department of Health and Social Security, 1987). Other policies have tried to achieve a much finer targeting at sub-regional levels. In the 1980s and 1990s they included the Healthy Cities Initiative, the Urban Programme, City Challenge and the Single Regeneration projects. In 1997 about a dozen Health Action Zones were designated by the government, all but two in the Midlands and north of England, and some £15 million was made available to them to tackle local causes of health inequalities and social deprivation (Jacobson and Yen, 1998).

Policies of this kind would, presumably, be seen by most people as fair, for they seek to equalize communities' access to health care in relation to their health needs, whatever their social or economic composition. They conform to the widely shared view that it is morally right to distribute health care resources in broad proportion to people's needs for them. And to the extent that the regions and zones with relatively high levels of need are also those with the largest concentrations of social and economic disadvantage, such policies may also effect a narrowing of the health gap, for any gains in health resulting from the expansion of services are likely to accrue in the least advantaged regions and zones. This was certainly in the mind of the government in creating the Health Action Zones, which were expected to 'provide a framework for the NHS, local authorities and other partners to work together to achieve progress in addressing the causes of ill health and reducing health inequalities' (Department of Health, 1997c, para. 4).

Justice and the narrowing of the health gap

Yet however just it may be to allocate the resources of the NHS broadly in proportion to the needs that communities have for them, there is no certainty that the same policies will also do very much to narrow the health gap, for the conventional indicators of morbidity and mortality at the population level are much more sensitive to socio-economic conditions beyond the control of the health service than they are to anything which is done by or within the service. As Benzeval has put it, 'the international evidence on inequalities in health is compelling. People who live in disadvantaged circumstances have more illnesses, greater distress, more disability and shorter lives than those who are more affluent' (Benzeval, Judge and Whitehead, 1995, p. xvii). The converse of this is that improvements in the quantity and quality of health care services have no very great impact on conventional indicators of poor health such as age-adjusted mortality rates (*op. cit.*, p. 95). The provision of more and better health services may go some way in this direction, but the well-springs of health inequalities cannot be plugged merely by building new hospitals and health centres or employing more health visitors and junior doctors.

If, then, policies for the redistribution of health care resources continue over time, the situation may eventually be reached in which the access that communities have to health care is broadly equal *in relation to their need*, whatever their level of social and economic deprivation, but in which the health gap stubbornly remains (Butler, 1979). One requirement of justice would then have been met: irrespective of their material conditions, people in different parts of the country would enjoy broadly similar levels of health care provision *relative to* their experiences of illness and death. Would it then be just to *continue* to redistribute the financial resources of the NHS in favour of the less well-off areas simply because of the persistence of a health gap which the NHS can do little more to close? Another way of putting essentially the same question is to ask whether it is right to use the resources of the NHS to compensate for broader social and economic ills if the effect of doing so is to discriminate against those living in more prosperous areas (New and Le Grand, 1996, p. 64). Provided people's access to health care at the level of the region, district or the health action zone is broadly proportional to their need for it, does justice in the allocation of health care resources require us to do anything more?

One answer could be yes: policies for the allocation of health care resources should continue to favour the less well-off areas or districts because, even if their continuing high levels of illness and death cannot much be changed by the NHS, they can at least be compensated by it. Justice, from this standpoint, requires not simply an *equal* access to health care in relation to need, but a *better* access in those places where, for whatever reasons, morbidity and mortality remain persistently high. But to argue in this way is to raise questions of justice for the more favoured regions and areas. Would it be justifiable actually to provide a *lower* level of access to care, relative to need, in better-off areas in order to provide the worse-off areas with a *higher* level of access? Do people living in the more favoured regions of the country have a moral claim for equal treatment, or can this justly be overridden in order to endow the less favoured regions with an appropriate compensation?

Narrowing the gap when resources are in short supply

The question assumes a sharper edge when resources are in short supply. In times of economic growth, when the money available for health care is increasing in real terms, it is easier to take a magnanimous view. The most disadvantaged regions and districts will receive the largest shares, but all will receive something. The process will be one of levelling up, not levelling down, and no region will actually be worse off. In times of recession, however, the picture will change. If the resources that are available for health care are increasing only very slowly (or, even worse, not at all), then any worthwhile redistribution to the less favoured places may only be achievable by *reducing* the amount of funding to those more favourably placed. It is not now a matter of giving some communities a smaller amount of growth money than others: it is a matter of actually reducing their existing levels of funding in order to release resources for redistribution elsewhere.

This, broadly, was the situation in England and Wales in the late 1970s, when the policy of revenue redistribution among the regions began to bite at precisely the time when the economy was slowing down and restraints on public spending were being imposed (Mays and Bevan, 1987). The result was that, among the better-off regions in the south-east of England (which under the policy of redistribution were receiving smaller allocations than those elsewhere), intra-regional reallocations in favour of the worst-off districts could be effected only by *cutting* the resources for the better-off ones. A reasonably clear distinction seems to be made in clinical medicine between withholding a treatment that has not yet begun and discontinuing one that is already in train. Ethically, the former appears to arouse less concern than the latter. Could a similar distinction be made in the allocation of resources? Is it ethically acceptable to reduce an *existing* level of service in order to switch resources to poorer communities?

Absolute and relative levels of health

Other possibilities can be imagined in which the narrowing of the health gap, however just it may be in principle, might nevertheless not be the right thing to do. One is suggested by Rawls' (1971) principle of difference: 'social and economic inequalities are to be arranged so that they are . . . to the greatest benefit of the least advantaged' (see Chapter 3). If 'health' is defined as a relevant inequality in this context, then the application of the principle of difference would justify increasing social inequalities in people's experiences of illness, disability and premature death *provided* they raised the absolute levels of health among those at the bottom of the pile. There is no necessary inconsistency between a widening of the health gap on the one hand and, on the other, an improvement in the health of those who are the least advantaged. Marmot and McDowell (1986) showed that, among British men aged between 20 and 64 in manual occupations, standardized mortality ratios (SMRs) for all causes of death, and for many major individual causes of death, fell between the early 1970s and the early 1980s. In *absolute* terms their health (to the extent that it was measured by their experience of early death) had improved over the ten-year period. However, because the SMRs of men in *non*-manual occupations had fallen by an even greater amount, their *relative* position had worsened. The same was true, though less marked, for married women aged between 20 and 54.

There are, of course, many possible explanations for such a striking set of results, some of which may be artefactual rather than substantive. The widening gap between the two occupational groups may have resulted either from significant changes in the classification of diseases over the period of the study or from changes in the definition of manual and non-manual occupations. Marmot and McDowell did not themselves attach much importance to such methodological possibilities. More probably, some of the social and behavioural factors which adversely affect mortality (and, conversely, some of the social and behavioural factors which protect against early death) had been differentially experienced by non-manual and manual workers. The former, for example, may have switched in greater numbers to diets that were low in saturated fats and high in fibre; more of them may have given up cigarette smoking; they may have experienced less unemployment; and their income levels may have risen more rapidly. Some combination of these possibilities would explain both the widening health gap reported by Marmot and McDowell and also the absolute improvement in SMRs among both non-manual and manual groups.

If this is a broadly correct interpretation, then it raises the interesting possibility that the widening gap between the SMRs of the non-manual and manual groups may simply have been the necessary price to be paid for improving the SMRs in *both* groups. A great deal and variety of publicity has been given over many years to the ways in which we can improve our chances of a long life, and all manner of campaigns have been mounted to persuade us to change our behaviour for the sake of our health. Let us assume, not unreasonably, that some of these messages have rubbed off onto a media-aware population that is well adapted to subliminal advertising. This would satisfactorily explain the absolute reductions in the SMRs of both groups. But let us also assume, equally reasonably, that the messages have been differentially perceived and acted upon and that they have had a greater impact among people in non-manual than in manual jobs. This would satisfactorily explain the widening gap in the SMRs. Are we then to say that the publicity should not have been dispensed and the change in behaviour should not have been urged because of the possible adverse impact on the health gap? Is it really more important to narrow the gap than it is to improve the health of the least advantaged? To argue that it is would seem to allow ideology to triumph over pragmatism.

The health gap could, moreover, be widened still farther if priority were to be given in the allocation of health care resources to services which deliver the greatest quantum of QALYs. Most league tables of costs per QALY show various preventive measures as offering good value for money: they are often cheap, and if they work they give good results in terms of both the quantity and quality of life extended. In Maynard's (1991) table, for example, cholesterol testing followed by dietary advice among people aged between 40 and 69 cost £220 per QALY at 1990 prices; advice from a GP to stop smoking cost £270; anti-hypertensive treatment among people aged between 45 and 64 cost £940; and cholesterol testing followed by drug treatment cost £1,480. (To set these figures in context, neurosurgery for malignant brain tumours cost £107,780 per QALY.) Investing in these kinds of preventive measures may well deliver large improvements in health among people across the whole spectrum of social division, but to the extent that they are taken up more enthusiastically by more advantaged sections of the population, the effect would be a widening in the health gap. Would such an eventuality be seen as a failure of health policy? And how much priority would the narrowing of the gap then have?

6

Stories from the coal-face

Collecting the stories

The purpose of telling stories

This chapter presents a number of 'stories' told by people in different positions in the NHS about their own experiences of rationing in health care and about the ethical issues to which they may – or may not – be seen to give rise. Telling stories has, in recent years, become an increasingly fashionable way of conveying information, arguing cases, and exploring the social world. This is as true in medical ethics as in many other areas of intellectual analysis (Nelson, 1997). Stories have an obvious and superficial appeal. They provide detail and texture; they show us the human face of abstract argument; and they allow us to peep into lives and experiences that may be very different from our own. We like stories because they entertain us and sustain us through the drier passages of whatever it is we are reading.

The uncritical telling of stories can, however, soon become a tedious and even a counter-productive affair. When the voyeuristic excitement has begun to fade, the question is left: so what? How has the story helped us to understand the point that it is illustrating? Indeed, why has the story-teller thought it worth telling the story at all? Such questions assume, if anything, an even greater complexity when they deal – or are presented as dealing – with issues that have a moral connotation. Are we supposed to read them as 'improving tales', instructing us in the rights and wrongs of the world? Are we to read them as 'cautionary tales', warning us of the gulf that all too often exists between the text-book accounts of ethical propriety and the blackguardly behaviour of real people? Or are we to read them simply as the narrative equivalents of the pictures in a book, illustrating the text in different ways in order to hold our interest and enlarge our understanding?

Answers to such questions need, it seems, to be given in each context in which the device of story-telling is deployed. Here, some tentative answers will be provided; but an understanding of the ways in which the stories in this chapter can be read is not easily separable from the means by which they were obtained. What follows, therefore, is first an account of how the stories came to be, and then some suggestions of how they can be read in the context of the book.

Methods

The idea of collecting and narrating some 'stories from the coal-face' began, quite simply, as an exercise in illumination. Some of the more abstract elements discussed in the foregoing chapters might, it was thought, be better understood through the use of illustrations drawn from the real lives of those who plan and deliver care in the NHS. Since the space available for these stories would be strictly controlled, no systematic attention was paid to their typicality. The aim was simply to collect a number of stories from workers occupying different professional roles in the service.

The first step was to ask colleagues in the NHS to recommend others who were known to them as thoughtful people who might be willing to tell their stories. A list of some 30 names resulted, spread across a number of different locations in the south of England. From this, 16 people were invited to take part in the study, the selection being guided mainly by the desire to include a diversity of professional roles. The letter of invitation contained a brief account of the study, together with a full explanation of the way in which the stories would be collected, analysed and used. The letter emphasized the control that each informant would have over his or her story at all stages. Of the 16 invitations sent, all but three were accepted.

In the second stage, those who had agreed to tell their stories were briefed about the topics they were intended to cover. The briefing emphasized that the topics were to be seen as an aid to structuring the conversation in certain areas, not as a formal set of questions to be answered. Some topics were likely to be more relevant than others, and some issues that were irrelevant to the informant's particular situation could be omitted altogether. The intention, it was explained, was to allow each story-teller to focus on the things that were important to him or her, and to talk about them in ways that were relevant to their particular experiences.

When the informants had had sufficient time to compose their ideas (usually two to three weeks), the author visited them and carried out a tape-recorded conversation. Since the statement of topics was not a questionnaire, each interview was different. Some informants spoke for long periods with little interruption from the author; others preferred the author to guide the conversation with regular questions. Most (but not all) came to the conversation with prepared notes, and these usually structured their ideas. Thirteen conversations were held, each lasting between about one and one-and-a-half hours, though two (with a health visitor and a district nurse) were later discarded because they duplicated other, more fruitful conversations.

The tape-recordings of the conversations were processed in two stages. Firstly, a straightforward transcript was made of each conversation, including the speech of both parties. Secondly, each transcript was edited by the author. Editing, in this context, had four objectives. The first was simply to render the spoken word, with all its grammatical and other imperfections, into readable text while preserving as much as possible of the original words and phrases. The second objective was to rearrange the disparate elements of the conversation, where necessary, into broad themes – though in fact the preparations that most informants had made prior to the conversations required fairly little of this to be done. The third objective of editing was to impose sense and meaning on things the informants had said where none had been apparent at face value, and the fourth was to strip the conversation of whatever clues might have led to the identification of the story-tellers.

Copies of the edited transcripts were then sent to each informant. In the full knowledge of how the stories were to be used, informants were asked to make any additions, deletions or corrections that they wished. The guarantees were repeated to them that any changes they wished to make would be accepted without question, and also that nothing would be done with the stories until the informants were entirely satisfied with them. In fact, the changes requested by the informants were, with only one exception, minor editorial amendments.

Methodological reflections

This way of gathering the stories has endowed them with some distinctive characteristics. They are, for example, likely to be reflective stories.

The informants had ample time to think about their ideas before each conversation and equally ample time after it to reflect upon (and change) what they had said. They retained full and absolute control over the contents of their stories and the ways their words were interpreted. The stories told here reflect precisely what their tellers want them to reflect. If some of them seem to veer towards the controversial or to reveal a hint of righteous indignation, it is because those who have told them wish them to be seen in such a way. The unusual but deliberate step of allowing the informants to read and freely change *anything* they wished in their narratives precludes any possibility of bias or distortion by the author.

But a reflective story is not necessarily a balanced one, and although the stories fairly reflect the intentions of their tellers, there is no reason to suppose that they were consciously trying to project an even-handed view of their work. Indeed, the very way in which the conversations were arranged, focusing as they did on the rationing of care, almost guarantees their bias. As the reader will discover, the informants concentrated largely on those areas of their work in which they were experiencing the greatest gaps between needs and resources. They did so because that is what they were asked to do – though some may have taken advantage of the opportunity to ride certain hobby-horses with particular vigour. We all like to complain, and the more interested and sympathetic the one upon whom we are venting our ire, the more pressingly our points may be made.

Nor, strictly speaking, are the stories representative of anything other than themselves. One surgeon's story cannot purport to be anything other than that – the story of one surgeon. To assume that it can stand in some sense for the collective experience of all surgeons – or even of all surgeons in the same hospital – is unwarranted. At the very least, however, the stories reveal the *kinds* of rationing that go on in the NHS and some of the *ways* they are handled by the front-line staff, even if they cannot give us any indication of their frequency. More than that, however, there may be a sense in which the stories are indicative, if not representative. Although no two surgeons will have exactly the same experiences, the lives of most surgeons must nevertheless have a good deal in common with each other. The general experiences of one are likely to find echoes in those of another, even though the details of their day-to-day work may differ. There is a risk that the *particular* people whose stories are told here were mavericks in extremely bad – or good – posts; but no such obvious extremes were known to the author, and whenever an informant was asked whether they thought it likely that their peers would tell similar stories, none identified his or her particular experience as obviously bleaker than others known to them.

The stories, moreover, encompass only a segment of the roles engaged in the rationing processes of the NHS. There are no stories from physiotherapists, junior nurses, speech therapists, chiropodists, dentists, radiographers, pharmacists and many others. There are no stories from patients. At best, then, the stories can give nothing more than a handful of selected insights into the rationing of care in the NHS, and nothing more is claimed for them. But how are we to read them in the context of an ethical discourse? What is the relationship between the moral positions adopted by those who were telling the stories and the possible ways in which we can think about an ethically defensible allocation of scarce resources for health care? The answer hinges around the view that we take of the assorted moral principles which the literature offers us about the fair, just and proper allocation of health care resources. Various positions, helpfully identified by Arras (1997), may be taken along a spectrum. At the risk of unwarranted simplification, three marker positions are considered here.

Ways of reading the stories

At one extreme, moral principles may be seen as having their own internal standing and legitimacy. They derive from informed moral reasoning, they attract a widespread sympathy, and they carry a weight of tradition, respect and acceptance. The principle of choosing between individuals in accordance with their needs might be one such principle (Chapter 2); so too might Doyal's (1995) specifications of a just distributional structure (Chapter 3). Such principles, for those who hold them, are largely non-negotiable; they are not available for modification in the light of whatever knowledge we might possess of how things actually work at the coal-face; they are not, in Doyal's graphic phrase, 'up for democratic grabs' (Doyal, 1997b, p. 178). For those who occupy this position on the spectrum, stories can never be more than a supplement to moral reasoning. They can illustrate the applications of moral principles in the hurly-burly of life at the coal-face and they can show the conditions under which — and the extent to which — practices are faithful to principles. But they cannot supplant or even modify the principles themselves. The stories are just that — stories. The behaviours which they reveal and the conditions which they expose may help us to see the extent to which certain principles are supported or threatened; but they do not interact with the principles themselves and they cannot change their substance.

In a middle position might be those who hold that, while moral principles are certainly weighty and enduring, they derive not just from abstract moral reasoning but also from the real conditions and the real experiences of real lives – and these are known mainly through the stories that people tell about them. Moral principles, from this perspective, are rooted in and develop out of the ways in which thoughtful and reflective people react to the moral puzzles that confront them. Morality grows out of social experience and social action, and as experience and action change and evolve, so too may the principles themselves. Stories, from this viewpoint, are more than simply an heuristic supplementation to external moral principles: they are the very stuff on which the principles are founded and out of which they evolve.

The occupants of this position on the spectrum will read the stories not only for whatever illumination they may cast on principles derived from moral reasoning above and beyond the variety of human behaviour, but also for the way in which the variety of human behaviour may test the principles themselves. These few humble stories will, of themselves, change nothing; but the insights they may give us into the ways in which thoughtful professional people are grappling with moral issues in their daily work may cause us to think again about the principles themselves. If the principled solution to a common problem becomes unworkable in circumstances that are commonly encountered in, say, the home nursing of elderly housebound patients, and if thoughtful and responsible nurses are tackling the problem from a different moral angle, this may affect the way we think about the principle. Ethical debate, from this perspective, is a creative organic activity, moving repeatedly between evidence and principle and allowing each to shape our judgments of the other. From this viewpoint the stories that people tell about their experiences become major sources of the evidence we require.

At an opposite extreme are those who stand in the emerging tradition of 'post-modern ethics'. Rejecting the possibility of any kind of grand coherence in our ethical views of the world, the post-modernist sees in the stories that people tell about their work neither a means of illuminating externally derived moral principles nor even a source of knowledge from which such principles can grow, but the principles themselves. Morality is as people do, and the small-scale narrative story – the *petit récit* – is actually the only way in which we can know about the morality of the real world. We each make a contribution to a moral understanding of the world around us by telling our stories: 'the idea of telling one's own story as a responsibility to the common-sense world reflects what I understand as the core morality of the post-modern' (Frank, 1995, p. 17).

Two consequences of some importance seem to follow from this.

Firstly, it becomes a matter of some importance *whose* stories get to be told. The bias in the stories that are narrated in this chapter thus becomes a bulky methodological impediment, for they have been chosen according to no defensible criteria. Secondly, the authenticity of the story-teller becomes as important as the ethical value of the story being told. Rogues and con-men are, presumably, as free to tell their story as are people of integrity and honesty; but to argue that all stories have an equal standing as a source of post-modern morality, whoever the teller may be, is to come close to the kind of moral nihilism that we rejected in Chapter 2. If, then, the stories in this chapter are read in a post-modern light, the professional probity of those who have told them becomes a matter of methodological relevance. In conducting the interviews, the author had no sense whatsoever of talking to the smattering of rotten apples that is to be found in any occupational barrel. Those who consented to tell their stories presented themselves as highly professional men and women of probity, commitment and compassion, trying to do the very best they could for their patients in the face of difficult odds. They were not paid for their co-operation; their conversations were thoughtful; and their actions were consistent with the altruistic motive of wishing to contribute to the betterment of human health.

Here, then, are three different ways in which the stories in this book can be read – and there are doubtless as many intermediate positions as readers may wish to construct for themselves. My readers must decide for themselves where they stand and read the stories accordingly. But under no circumstances should too much be read into them. For all the reasons rehearsed above, they constitute a miniscule selection of black-and-white snapshots taken (if the metaphor will bear it) with a Brownie camera. They come no closer than that to the multi-coloured wide-screen movie with wrap-around sound that we would ideally like to be viewing about the rationing processes of the NHS.

The stories

The health visitor's story

Most of the work I do is with children with special needs, and there are not many of us doing this kind of work locally. This makes it an almost impossible job because there are hundreds of children in the area with special needs. My workload now has become excessive, and I'm having to decide which jobs are the most important. I'm having to prioritize. What happens is that if a consultant refers a child to me or if a parent rings in,

I do my own assessment; and if it seems an inappropriate referral, such as a school-aged child with very minimal needs, I will try and pass it on down the line to the school nurses or the ordinary health visitors. But if it's a new-born baby with a disability, or one who is diagnosed with cerebral palsy, then it's my priority. I start with them. I usually always do a home visit first, to carry out my own assessment, and then as I'm sitting there I decide whether it is something I'm to keep or whether it's something I am going to pass on to someone else. It's all down to my own assessment.

I don't have a budget and I'm not dishing out any particular treatments or equipment myself, so that kind of rationing doesn't come into it. But rationing that happens somewhere else has a knock-on effect on my work. I may be visiting a family where a child has complex physical needs and requires some equipment. The money for it comes from social services; and if the budget for that equipment is rationed, it affects what I can do. I can't move forward with that family until they get the equipment they need. It really impacts on the health of a family if they can't get a special piece of equipment or a special potty chair because their child has, say, cerebral palsy. They then become the victims of rationing decisions that have been taken elsewhere and over which I have no control. Much of my work is on the bridge between social and health care. What is hard for me is that because I'm the key person to co-ordinate things, these failures land up on my desk. Neither side accepts responsibility and I'm caught in the middle.

For instance, if you have a child with a social communication disorder, then one of the first things you try to do is to get him into something like an ordinary playgroup. But to do that he would need the support of another person and there's no funding for it. That comes under social services. To my mind it's a very simple thing that should happen very quickly, but there's often no money for it. Actually I call it discrimination because children are entitled to go to playgroup from two-and-a-half years; but children with social communication disorders aren't being assessed for this kind of funding until they are three. So they are being discriminated against. They don't have the same rights as other children. I get quite angry about it.

Another effect of the shortage of resources is that there's only one person employed to do my job. If a family needs special support while I'm on holiday or off sick, there's no cover for me. So the service stops. And you think well, why have we got this wonderful intensive service if it comes to a halt just because I'm not around? We did suggest bringing all the paediatric nursing services together as a team, so that even if somebody was on holiday or off sick we could still provide a continuous service for our families and someone would always be there at the end of the phone. But the powers-that-be are still discussing it!

It's the same with the early referral of children with developmental delays. The whole idea now is to identify these children as early as possible. When the community paediatrician diagnoses a child with, say, a social communication disorder or autism she'll ring me up within 48 hours and I will see the family within a week to try and get some services mobilized. But of course there are very limited resources to meet the needs of these kinds of children; and I seriously wonder why we are identifying them and sending the specialist health visitor in so early because it only encourages the parents to expect something to happen. All right, I can go in and I can talk to them and I can listen and support them emotionally, but at the end of the day they want some action; yet because resources are very limited, nothing may happen for quite a while. The whole idea of identifying children with social communication problems is that the earlier you can get some intervention in there, the more progress these children are going to make. So you get frustrated because you can't always say to the parents, look, we could help your child but I'm afraid there isn't much we can do for the time being.

And then again, sometimes services seem to be limited or rationed but it may just be that they're simply inaccessible to the patients who need them. I suppose it is rationing by inaccessibility. Services can be so hard to get at. They're there somewhere, but you just can't mobilize them for your patients. Everything is so complex even in this little area, and if I can't access them, God help these poor families who have to climb over so many hurdles to get there. For instance, recently I needed to get a laundry service for a family. It should have been a simple matter of dealing with colleagues in the community services – phoning them, say – but oh no!, it took about two weeks before this bit of paper arrived on my desk authorizing the service for the family. And that, I think, is rationing because if you put up enough hurdles, the demand for that service will fall off. People just won't bother, even though they really need it at that particular time. And the sad thing is that the people who are going to be most put off won't be the well-educated middle-class families who understand the system. It will be the poor families, under-educated, inarticulate. They're the ones who suffer most. Rationing doesn't work fairly. It's biased.

From my past experience I think that many health visitors would say the same. They're doing as much as they possibly can, and they're very frustrated. How do you cope with it? Well you just get on, don't you? You just cope because you have to. But I do think it's detrimental to your emotional well-being. Sometimes it affects you very badly – particularly if you're working with a family that has been pulled apart, who need something to support them, who need a piece of equipment or some kind of service or help or something. It's not like hospital nursing: you haven't isolated that family and put it in a hospital. They're not in a clinical situation where you can detach yourself from them and become emotionless. You get used to doing that when you're a nurse, but this is a real family living in a real home in the real world. That's why it's harder.

Of course I realize that there is only a certain amount of money to go around, but I do think that learning disabilities and physical and mental disabilities are all very low priority areas in all the services – not just in health, but in education and social services too. It's not like major heart surgery: everyone sees that that's really exciting and they want to plough money into it. Disabled children are a very low priority. They have never had loads of money poured into them. But it's very short-sighted. There's almost no higher priority than getting children to become as independent as early as they can and to develop their characters as fully as they can. It must be an investment. If we can get these children to be as independent as possible, then they won't be using the services as much later on in their lives. And it's not only the child. If the services aren't there, and if you're not relieving some of the family stress by supporting them in helping their child, there's a knock-on effect to the family's own physical and mental health. And if the family breaks down, then that will cause more problems later down the line.

Time is also a precious commodity. If a family is given a diagnosis or a baby is born with Down's syndrome, that family needs a huge amount of time – ideally you need to be available maybe twice a week, maybe every other day to start with. It's not going to go on like that for ever, but it is for the first few days and weeks. But I often find I have to wean the parents off me before they're really ready to be on their own simply because I have to move on to the next family. It shouldn't happen – they're bereaved. Parents who have got a new diagnosis go through a bereavement. It's as simple as that. You sit there and you see it week after week, day after day. While you're in with those families it takes up a huge amount of my time. I have to drop everything else and you just don't know when the next one is coming up. So if two or three families are going through this sort of crisis at the same time it takes chunks out of my time; and then I have to cut down on all the other things that I would be doing. So yes, I would definitely say that I have to consciously restrict the time I spend with families in real need. And this is cutting down the quality of the care, isn't it, because listening and talking things over is an essential part of the care and treatment I can give them.

It all comes back to priorities. Mine as well as society's. And of course it's very difficult sometimes to make the choices. I will always try to give priority to children who have got the most severe need or where I know I can make a difference. I'll invest more time in them than other families where I know I'm not going to make very much difference. That's the way I ration in my head, you know. If I've got to divide my time between two families, I'll give most of it to the family where I think I'll make the most progress rather than the family where I know I'm going to bang my head against a brick wall. But then I think, gracious, that's a dreadful thing to do. It may not be wrong, but it's definitely discrimination. That's the reality of it, it's discrimination. Maybe it's based on ethnicity. Or it may be that I can move that family ahead more quickly because there isn't a language barrier. Or maybe it's a cultural or a social class factor. Perhaps poverty is the sticking-point. And that's discrimination. I make these calculations quickly in my head, instinctively really, and that's the fact of it. When I look back and reflect on what I do, I can see that it's discrimination, but that's reality.

It's not really a conscious thing, though. I don't really think about why I'm investing time in this family and not that one. It doesn't work as neatly as that. All you think is, right, I can do that and I'll get a result and then I can sort out someone else's problems later on. But maybe you'll never get around to them. I never actually think of myself as making judgments like that, but subconsciously I must be. All you think is, here's a family that normally functions very well, but they've fallen apart and I must do something about it. And then there are other families that haven't been functioning well at all and you think, well, a few more weeks won't make any difference. It's not a matter of judging whether one set of criteria is more important than another. There aren't any criteria. I couldn't really tell you how I make these decisions. You just do, don't you? But you may be discriminating. Just recently, for instance, I've had quite a few families where English is not the first language and where they've had children diagnosed as severely delayed in their social and language development; and now I reflect on it, yes, I have spent less time with them. They're limited with their language and they can't talk very much about their problems, so I do less listening and talking. It's not fair to them. They probably need me more than most. So yes, things like social class and race and language all play a part in how much care you give people.

I think it would be better for rationing decisions in the health service to be much more open and honest. It's far too much like the secret service. After all, it is a public service and we should all know where we stand. I suppose that if anyone has to make the decisions, it should be the workers who are dealing with the everyday reality of the service. If you leave it to the managers, well, the higher up the decision-makers are, the more out of touch they are with what really happens. What needs to happen is that, when something can't be done for a family because you haven't got the time or you haven't got the money or the equipment isn't there, there should be a proper way of documenting the deficiency and it should be clear who the document is going to and what they must do with it. So that if I go into a family and there's something that I can't do for them, I should be able to put it down very clearly on a formal sheet of paper and the family should know where it's going. At least it would help me to feel better because I would know that it wasn't my fault; and the family might possibly feel a little better as well because they would know that someone in authority was looking at the problem.

There should then be a management response, and from that the service can develop. The managers must either say, there's a real problem here and we must find a way of responding to it, or else they must say, we recognize that there's a problem but we haven't got any money for it – it's not a service that we're providing at the moment. If they did this, we would at least know exactly where we stood. As it is, we have meeting after meeting after meeting just to keep discussing the problems. Managers are afraid to change the way you work in case it upsets somebody. It's management caution and political inertia and all of those things. Red tape. Bureaucracy. A lot of resources are wasted, really. Myself, I would go for the jugular, I'm that sort of person; but managers, or certain managers, say oh no, we've got to do it drip, drip, drip, much more slowly. I know a lot of people would think I'm being idealistic. They think I want too much for the families. But I don't think I'm being idealistic. It's common sense really. If a family falls apart, and their physical and mental and emotional health breaks down, it will cost the country far more to pick up the pieces. But no, managers don't look that far ahead.

We also need to find ways of giving patients a proper part to play in the rationing process. At the moment, patients in the NHS don't get a say at all, do they? They're made to think they should be grateful for whatever service they're getting, however lousy it is. So if you try and get them to complain about it, or if you say they really ought to write to the health authority because it's not good enough, they won't do it. They're just grateful for what they're given. Obviously there are some people who do complain and stand up for themselves, but in general I don't think people do. I try to say to them, well, actually it's a service that you are entitled to and you have paid for. But they can't see it like that.

It's partly that children with special needs are forgotten. Caring for these children doesn't involve fancy treatments or require expensive equipment. It hasn't got the same glamour attached to it as a special care baby unit. There's a lot of medical wizardry in the hospital, a lot of attention and a lot of money going into it. It's back again to priorities, and children with special needs quite simply have a low priority. They get a rough deal when it comes to sharing out the resources. That's the culture. That's how it is. I think we're changing, though, and in time we'll shift a little bit further away from the awe in which we hold modern medicine. Eventually services for families and community-based services will acquire a much higher priority. We've just to keep standing on our soapboxes and raise the profile of children with disabilities and special needs. In time it may have a knock-on effect, but nothing's going to happen overnight.

The surgeon's story

The rationing that I see is not something that happens when managers sit around a table and ask whether the health service can reasonably afford this procedure or that one, or whether some of the things that the service has traditionally provided are no longer to be within the pale. Of course, I'm not saying that this sort of thing doesn't happen at all, but the rationing that I see in my work is done on an entirely haphazard and unplanned basis – almost on a minute-by-minute basis depending on whether the facilities are there at the particular moment when you need them. Rationing as I encounter it is unplanned. It's not purposeful. It happens simply because something that ought to be there isn't there. Sometimes it happens by accident, sometimes because no care plan has been put into place, sometimes because someone has failed to make a decision. That's the sort of rationing that I come up against. It's most definitely *not* rationing in the sense of deciding that we are not going to do such-and-such an operation on patients of such-and-such an age because the outlook for them is so poor or because they've brought it on themselves.

As clinicians, we're having to make continual decisions as we go along about what care our patients are going to receive. But I think to call it implicit rationing is to give a rather fancy name to what is a completely haphazard and *ad hoc* process. Something will be rationed one day but not the next, and whether it is rationed or not will depend on something as tenuous as the day of the week or the month of the year. It happens on an almost random basis. Sometimes it's predictable and sometimes it's not. When it is predictable, then I suppose you must say that yes, it is implicit rationing. When it's not predictable, either because of a lack of foresight or bad luck, then I think to call it implicit rationing is perhaps rather overstating the case. And it affects different investigations at different times. At the moment there's a six-month wait for an MRI [magnetic resonance imaging] scan whereas last year you waited six months for a barium enema. So these things happen as you go along. They've not been planned, and when the problem has been there for long enough, and enough people have complained, somebody eventually produces some extra sessions which miraculously manage to clear the backlog.

But you have to realize that the really expensive part of the health service isn't the treatment but the investigations that we do. They're the things that really cost money, not only because of the cost of the tests themselves but also the time spent hanging around waiting for the tests to be done and then waiting for the results. It really is a fearfully expensive exercise. We saw this with the introduction of CT [computed tomography] scanning. When we bought the latest CT scanner out of money raised by public subscription, the clinicians all agreed in advance that we would be very selective about using it. A scan would only be done in limited circumstances and with the explicit approval of a consultant. But of course the reality is quite different from this, and everyone now has a CT scan for everything. The slightest headache is likely to end up with one because you are terrified that someone might have a cerebral tumour. So even if you really intend to use a facility reasonably and rationally, you find that the practical politics are different; and of course, the more people who use a test, the longer they have to wait for it to be done. You get a queue developing, and if a patient suddenly has an urgent need for a scan, then either people have to be pushed aside or it doesn't get done.

This is what's happening now with MRI scanning. People are having to wait for up to six months for an MRI scan. You might try to get a scan for a patient with a potential malignancy, only to discover that women are having MRI scans to see whether their breast prostheses have leaked. You do have to wonder about priorities! What usually happens is that you arrange an investigation for a patient, and then a week or two later the patient telephones to complain or grumble that they are having to wait two or three months for it to be done. What are we going to do about it? Could it be speeded up? Could they have it done privately? And when that happens, you obviously do try to speed things up. But the next time you see someone with the same condition, you wonder whether that particular investigation is absolutely essential. You know that there's a longish wait for it, so you might decide not to do it at all or else to do another test where there's a shorter wait. Sometimes you might put the whole thing off until the next time you see the patient.

So yes, when patients ring up and they sound rather irate and they ask what's happening, you try to get something done. That's how it works – very much so – but the unfortunate result is that people who push and shove a bit will get the best treatment. What worries me is that it's largely related to their social class. If you're upper middle-class, shall we say, and you've been told you have to wait six weeks for an MRI scan, then you know how to throw your weight around a bit. You know how to make a fuss. You know that if you ring up the secretary every day for a week, she will eventually cave in and make another arrangement. But the little old lady in social class four will simply say oh well, that's how things are, I've got to wait. So there is always likely to be an imbalance in who gets what simply because some people know how to manipulate the system. It doesn't happen all the time, but that's how it works when it does.

Apart from the routine pre-operative tests, most of the tests that we do are done to exclude cancer, so you only know in retrospect whether it was terribly urgent or not. And of course by the nature of things only a very small proportion of the cancer tests we do actually turn out to be positive. If it is cancer, you then have to make up your mind how urgent it's going to be; and if you think that early treatment is going to make a difference to the outcome, then you have to ring up one of the radiologists and take some special initiative to overcome the backlog which you know is there. Sometimes, of course, you don't know that there is a backlog, and it's not until people start complaining that you become aware of the problem. I wouldn't say it's a major problem, but it does seem to be one which is inherent to the health service.

But we must keep it in perspective. Yes, there are times where these delays make a real difference to the patient, but they are few and far between. Usually you know if there is going to be a delay and you know if the patient is anxious. More often than not you get it right. But you can't keep a mental note in your head of the waiting list for every test that's done in the hospital, particularly those which you don't request very often or which you haven't done for a long time. So if you ask me how long an abdominal CT scan will take, the answer is 'I don't know'. If you ask me how long an abdominal ultrasound test will take, I do know that it's far too long – two or three months. Certainly if I had an abdominal pain and I was told I needed an abdominal ultrasound, I would go away and have it done somewhere else, because I am not prepared to wait three months. So because I know that the wait for abdominal ultrasound is unacceptably long, I may not even request it. Or if I was particularly keen to have this test done, I may ring up the radiologist and explain the urgency and try to arrange an early date. But it doesn't happen very often. When you work in the health service you become aware of the constraints, and by and large you manage to work around them. Things don't always turn out exactly as you would like them to do, but the times when the patient suffers anything more than inconvenience or delay or anxiety are quite rare, though they do happen. In very extreme cases the result may be a loss of life.

On the whole, delays of this kind apply only to tests and investigations, not to treatments. I very rarely have to make *ad hoc* rationing decisions about treatments. But having said that, there are some situations where it does happen. Some of them are what I would call marginal procedures – those which don't affect the patient's life-span. I'm thinking of the removal of tattoos and the reversal of sterilization and that sort of thing. A great deal of energy is wasted discussing the costs and ethics of these procedures. But there are others that we *should* be talking about, where the constraints are so serious that people aren't actually talking about them, or if they are talking about them, not an awful lot is happening. I'm thinking of things like coronary artery surgery, renal failure in the elderly and pacemakers.

I don't myself encounter any of these, but one that I do come across from time to time is acute vascular surgery – aortic aneurysms that are leaking. Patients who are admitted as emergencies will invariably die if they are not operated on within an hour or two. But because a leaking abdominal aneurysm is relatively uncommon, it's simply not possible to have a specialist vascular surgeon on duty in every district general hospital every day of the week. That is why attempts are now being made to concentrate vascular surgery in a smaller number of acute hospitals where the expertise can be made available. But if a specialist *isn't* available, then patients with aortic aneurysms will be operated on by general surgeons who have not been well trained to do the procedure and who won't achieve as good an outcome as the specialists. So there's a dilemma. Do we train lots of vascular surgeons who then haven't got enough to do, or do we concentrate four or five of them on one site and require all emergency cases to go there? It's a kind of rationing. A patient with this particular diagnosis may not be getting the best care, although the problem is likely to be the non-availability of a specialist surgeon rather than a lack of resources or operating theatres or intensive care.

As a rule, of course, you should never admit defeat. You should always try to do something, however much it might cost and however unpromising the outcome. But you can't entirely ignore the costs. To operate on a patient over 80 with an aortic aneurysm and other concomitant problems such as high blood pressure and poor renal function would be costly not only in terms of the theatre but also of the intensive care unit during the week before the patient – in all probability – dies. In this situation, I think that many vascular surgeons would take the view that the chances of a successful outcome are so low and the patient's quality of life is so poor that to operate would not be an appropriate use of resources. It's not *only* a question of resources, however; it's also about the dignity of the patient and his family if he is put through a major operation, with all that this entails, before succumbing. It's a very difficult value judgment, but yes, there are emergency situations in which you decide to withhold treatment and allow the patient to die in dignity because the expected outcome is so poor.

It's different with waiting lists. In my own specialty, patients very rarely die on the waiting list. The rare situations where this happens are those that we have already talked about – people with aneurysms who are waiting for surgery. But it must be more common in cardiac surgery even though I can't actually quote you chapter and verse. One area which does concern me, even though it's not in my immediate experience, is angina. If, shall we say, my wife presents to her general practitioner with a lump in her breast, then she will be seen by a breast specialist within ten days, she will have tests done on the day she attends the clinic, she will be given the results of the test that day, and if she needs to have an operation she will be admitted within a fortnight. On the other hand, if I have a pain in my chest and I think I've got angina, I may have to wait a year to see a cardiologist and another year to have a cardiac angiogram. If it transpires that I need to have an operation, I may wait a further year for it. As a matter of equity there does seem to be a bit of a credibility gap here that reveals a real issue about rationing.

Why this happens, of course, is that the cardiac surgeon has nothing to do with breast cancer and the breast surgeon has nothing to do with heart disease, and there is no co-ordination between the different services. There are no cross-linkages that would enable us to prioritize either the speed or the order at which patients are seen in different specialties. If there's going to be any kind of co-ordination, it must be hatched at the top of the policy tree, for there would be long-term implications for things like the training of cardiac surgeons and the funding of cardiology centres. This obviously does occur to some extent, but I suspect there is much more political mileage in providing instant services for breast cancer than for angina, and it's also much cheaper. If a worried woman gets an out-patient appointment and it turns out that she hasn't got breast cancer, she has got her reassurance at the cost of nothing more than an examination and a test. But a cardiological investigation and a coronary angiogram are very specialized and highly expensive. So yes, of course there are resource constraints: coronary artery disease doesn't seem to have a high priority in non-emergencies.

It also comes back to what we were talking about a moment ago – the class factor. It's a matter of real concern to me that the poorest people in the community seem to have the worst health and the highest mortality, and we don't seem to be able to do very much to correct it. Obviously to an extent it has to do with things like smoking, but nevertheless it does appear to be the poorest sectors of the population that have the worst outcomes. They are disadvantaged at almost every turn, and we have a large responsibility towards them. I think to a certain extent that they should actually be targeted with extra resources. What we must avoid at all costs is making moralistic judgments about them. The question is often raised of whether perhaps we should avoid operating on people who seem to be bad hats; but that doesn't enter into our judgment at all. If anything, it's the other way around and we go out of our way to look after the disadvantaged. If the well-to-do and upper-class patients then start complaining that they're being kept waiting in the out-patients, they'll probably go privately anyway – not that they're kept waiting on purpose.

There is another and unfortunately much more frequent situation where the standard of care is less than satisfactory and this occurs when patients who are booked for elective surgery turn up at the right place and the right time only to find that there is no bed available for them. They may be scheduled for an operation at 9.00 in the morning and they're asked to come at 7.30; but at 8.50 they're still sitting out in the hall with all their relatives. They've not been interviewed, their consent has not been obtained, and they've had no pre-medication. They don't know whether they're going to be sent home or whether they're going to the operating theatre. And then sometimes a bed suddenly becomes available and they're given ten minutes' notice of the arrival of the theatre trolley. It's all too easy in that kind of situation for a lot of safety issues to get swept aside in the rush – making sure that they have had a pre-medication, that their consent has been taken, that the site of the operation has been marked, and that their last food and drink intake has been recorded. Fortunately it's very unusual for this to be fundamentally deleterious to patients. And in terms of rationing, they will get their operations eventually – maybe next week or next month. Sometimes they do get them straight away, even though it may all have been done in a slightly rushed and undignified way without the safety features which you would like to see in place. But it then becomes an issue about quality rather than rationing.

The pressure at which we sometimes have to work can also adversely affect the quality of our care. It's a quality issue which goes right through the day. You've got really too much to get through in the day. You're trying to do too much in the 24 hours. And it means that some patients don't get as much of your time as they would like. You may have done whatever is necessary for their proper care; but they nevertheless feel that they've had short change from you because you're in a hurry and they don't like to ask you a question. That doesn't happen so much in the out-patient clinics but it does happen on the wards. I might arrive in the morning to find either three patients admitted overnight or 30 patients. If there are 30 and I'm on duty, I feel I've got to see them. So the patients may get a rushed or less-than-thorough service.

So a major impact of rationing in my sphere is lack of time – always trying to get a quart out of a pint pot. Everything is a rush and a scramble, and these are not things that are decided by sitting around the table in a democratic way and discussing the ethics of rationing – they're just how things are. And it's all been compounded by the ageing of the population and the rising expectations of patients and their relatives. The increasing use of deputizing services and the reductions in GPs' hours have increased the numbers of patients being admitted to hospital, and the difficulties in discharging them are no longer confined to the acute medical patients. More of them now are also acute surgical patients. So the physicians are overwhelmed and the accident and emergency department is desperately overcrowded, not only in my hospital but throughout the health service. I don't think anybody really understands why this has happened.

My personal view is that not only has the population got older but it's also got iller. Unfortunately this is happening at precisely the time the government is reducing the number of hospital beds and putting more and more emphasis on day surgery; and as a result, elective surgery has gone to the back burner. And there's an important paradox here: the waiting list initiative and the drive for day surgery have tended to maximize the amount of inappropriate or unnecessary or inessential surgery that we now find ourselves doing. It's easier now to get your varicose veins operated on than it is to have your gall bladder removed, because there's a maximum time that patients are allowed to wait for the operation on their veins and it can be done as a day case. So we say, we'll get a locum to do the veins on a Saturday morning because that way we'll clear a chunk of the waiting list at relatively small cost.

But if you need in-patient surgery you may find yourself waiting for much longer than if you've got a pimple or a wart or something rather unimportant to be operated on. Patients with colorectal cancer, for example, are waiting a long time to be seen because it's become a specialist procedure and there simply aren't enough specialists. In a sense, they are the victims of the endless endoscopies, varicose veins, tonsils, grommets, and other such things that are still done in large numbers. So I don't see very much ethics in the rationing that actually goes on. I see a shortage of beds and of time and I find myself trying to cope with the increased demand within those constraints.

The problem is compounded by the inappropriate use of hospital beds. People cannot come into hospital for an operation or as an emergency if there are no beds available for them, yet we know from the evidence from this hospital and many others both in the US and the UK that a third of acute hospital beds are used inappropriately on any one day of the week, most particularly on Saturdays and Sundays. There are many reasons for this, including the lack of less intensive facilities elsewhere in the community, the lack of care plans, the lack of planned patient discharges, and the attitude of patients who don't want to go home or whose relatives cannot collect them. And then there are delays in waiting for test results which were done several days earlier, ward rounds which get delayed, transport difficulties, and delays in arranging rehabilitation. People now must have a care plan before they are discharged from hospital, and this has been a good thing; but it has undoubtedly had its down side in terms of keeping people in hospital longer than they really need to be. And that means that other people are kept out. And sometimes surgeons who fear that a bed will not be available on the day they're going to operate will block one by admitting the patient prematurely or keeping the existing occupant in longer than is necessary.

In other words there is a rationing of resources because people are staying in hospital longer than they need to, and this is one of the problems of a monopoly health service in which doctors spend the whole of their working life. The simple fact is that it doesn't make any difference to them or to the patient sitting in front of them whether they go home today or tomorrow. It's very interesting to see that in the private sector, hospitals are now employing fairly high-calibre nursing staff to harass consultants to get the patients out. They will ring you up on a daily basis and ask whether Mrs X is going home tomorrow or today. Is there any reason why she shouldn't go today? What's the problem? Is there anything I can do to help? Yes, of course I can arrange transport for her. This afternoon? Certainly. That's how it's done. I've tried to introduce that kind of approach in this hospital with, I have to say, very limited success. People get enthusiastic for a few weeks but then it evaporates.

The commissioning manager's story

Rationing is a heavily laden term and people have differing inter-
pretations. If you define rationing as 'care that would have been given if
the resources had been available', it assumes that services are explicitly
withheld because the money or the resource aren't there. I'm not
absolutely sure that this is the case, because although I can think of many
instances in my work in the health authority where we take decisions on
priorities, there are relatively few instances where patients are denied
treatment full stop. (There are some and I'll talk about those in a
moment.) Rather, what the health service tends to do, particularly in
secondary care, is to say well, you *can* have your operation, but you will
have to wait 18 months for it. It *will* be provided, but when and how it
will be provided are affected by resource constraints. I think clinicians,
particularly consultant surgeons, are able to make their own distinctions,
based upon the clinical indications as to what must be done quickly,
between cases that are urgent and those which can wait. If you want to
call that rationing, then fine; but I would call it prioritizing. I don't want
to get drawn into the fact that the government won't accept that
rationing exists in the health service. It clearly does, but to my mind it's
more about doctors making judgments about clinical priorities.

There are, however, instances where, in my experience in this health
authority and others, decisions do have to be made that a service will not
be provided to certain patients. The example that everyone always uses is
treatment for sub-fertility. This health authority, along with most others
I think, does purchase some sub-fertility services, but only for patients
who satisfy certain criteria about age, the stability of their relationship,
the children they have had from previous relationships, and so on. If as a
patient you don't satisfy those criteria, then this health authority will not
buy that service for you. This does seem to me to be an explicit rationing
decision. It's yes or no. Similarly in plastic surgery we have a protocol
which says that you will receive NHS treatment for, say, breast reduction
if you satisfy certain physiological preconditions. If you don't, then this
health authority will not pay for your operation. That again is a clear
example of a rationing decision, and it is made against a clear set of
criteria, one of which is financial. In other words, the health authority has
taken the view that because its resources are finite, it doesn't want to buy
a certain set of operations unless its criteria are satisfied. This is where
resource constraints may enter the picture. If the health authority had
unlimited resources, or even ten times the money that we actually have,
then I am pretty certain that its criteria for access to sub-fertility services
would be more relaxed than they are at the moment.

My experience is that rationing decisions of this sort are made in a relatively *ad hoc* way. No government has actually told the health authorities which services they can commission and which they can't. I think myself that the present government is beginning to walk down that particular road with things like national service frameworks and priority areas. Only today there has been an announcement on mental health which is clearly indicating the things that health authorities should be buying. I think the reason why services like sub-fertility treatment and cosmetic surgery are subject to criteria for access while, say, hernia repairs are not, is that they are seen as marginal services over which the health authority has some discretionary choice. Sub-fertility is something about which health authorities perceive they have a choice, whereas hernia repairs or varicose veins – rightly or wrongly – are not seen by health authorities in the same way. There is, I think, a traditional core of standard work that has always gone on in the district general hospital, and it's seen as no business of the health authorities to query whether it should change.

I suppose a lot of it is about convenience rather than life-and-death issues. Although much of what goes on in a standard district general hospital doesn't involve any great risk of mortality or even of long-term morbidity, nevertheless services such as sub-fertility and plastic surgery are different. The failure to provide them may cause considerable distress and the result may be a great deal of inconvenience to patients, but it isn't going to affect their health status. They are not going to suffer long-term morbidity as a result of not receiving that treatment. Actually, I would qualify that by saying that there *are* instances where the health authority explicitly allows its protocols and its criteria to be overridden. An example would be the case of breast reduction where genuine psychological distress is being caused or where the woman is suffering other illnesses or disabilities or pain associated with her condition. These need to be alleviated, and if the only way to alleviate them is through surgery for breast reduction, then it doesn't matter that it may not strictly be justified by the protocol. The way it would work in this health authority is that, under the protocol, the plastic surgeon would have to clear the operation with the authority before he could carry it out, and this would be done through a discussion between the surgeon and our consultant in public health medicine who specializes in this area. It's very much along the lines of the old extra-contractual referrals.

The basic protocol defining what would and would not be funded in plastic surgery was put together by the officers of the health authority on the basis of practice up and down the country. We then discussed it with the local plastic surgeons and GPs. This was at a time when primary care was becoming more important in the NHS and we had to get the GPs involved in explicit decisions about priorities. Then we took it to the health authority for a decision. They had to be the final arbiter because there was a major conflict between what the plastic surgeons wanted to do and what the GPs felt was appropriate. It may not have been right to place so much emphasis on the views of the GPs because they are not always the best judges of right and wrong; and in this case there was a very clear disagreement between them and the plastic surgeons about what was cosmetic and what wasn't. So in the end it was the health authority, having sought the advice of its officers, that had to take a decision on where the line would be drawn.

Of course there is an argument that there may be some services which the NHS has traditionally provided in the past, but which we can no longer afford to include in the core of the state-funded service. If people want to have them that's fine, but they will have to pay for them privately. I think the difficulty with such an argument is that it clearly runs counter to all that is currently being said at the national level, particularly by this government, about the availability of care that is free at the point of access. It seems to me that it would be very difficult to reach anything like a meaningful consensus about what should be in the core and what should not, and it would be very risky, politically, to try to make the distinction. Rather, I would go along with the government's view that it really is possible to provide a modern and adequate – indeed good – national health service from public funds that meets most of the needs of most of the people within a reasonable period of time. Of course, it requires a strength of purpose at the national level, particularly in fundamental things like resource allocation. The government must commit itself to growth in the health service of roughly 3 per cent a year in real terms, and there's evidence that this government, at least, is doing that. And then within that, the health authorities must enter into discussions with clinicians and user groups and others about the criteria that should determine people's access to the universally provided services.

An example of what I have in mind would be revascularization for the over-80s: artery bypass grafts and angioplasties to restore the blood flow to the heart where there is coronary heart disease. These are very effective operations and there's very good evidence that they work not only to increase life expectancy but also to restore the patient's quality of life. It's one of the few operations where the health service can put its hand on its heart – no pun intended! – and say this is a good thing and we should be doing more of it. But there is a debate in cardiology at the moment, both locally and I think internationally, about the circumstances in which access to bypass grafts and angioplasties might be denied to certain people because they are too old. It's not that they couldn't benefit from these operations, or that the operations couldn't be done on older people: it's simply that, in an environment where resources are tight, elderly patients are not the priority. To put it bluntly, we are edging towards a debate about whether people of 80 or more should be offered revascularization. It's not a debate that is local to us: it could be happening in Norfolk or Manchester or anywhere else, and it's a debate about whether we should be giving priority in our use of resources to the treatment of younger patients.

This is, of course, a very difficult area, and it's one that I think the government would prefer us to avoid; but nonetheless it's certainly a debate that's going on within cardiology. What is more, there are disagreements within cardiology about the way in which a patient's capacity to benefit from expensive operations like revascularization can be measured. You can draw up a system of scoring the benefits that patients will get from the procedures, but you are still left with the question of where you draw the cut-off. Do you say that everyone with a score above 10 on a scale from 1 to 15 will receive the treatment and everyone below 10 will not, or do you decide some other cut-off point? And do you keep shifting the line according to the amount of money that's available to deliver the service? This is very much a real debate at the moment.

I think one important implication of all of this is that we may be seeing some kind of limitation on clinical freedom. Of course I am well aware that doctors and nurses have always been making their own decisions about who gets what and in what circumstances. Those are rationing decisions taken by clinicians working on the basis of their judgment and experience. What I am saying, I think, is that within this there may be a role for more explicit protocols or guidelines about who gets what and in what circumstances. The important thing is that these kinds of decisions about where the line is to be drawn are not ones that the professionals should be making on their own. They are decisions for all the agencies involved in them. Yes, professionals are clearly one of the principal partners, but there is also a role for health authorities, patients themselves and even for the government in deciding where the cut-off point will lie. And that, I think, is a huge leap in thinking for the medical profession. There is perhaps now an opportunity, in cardiology and in one or two other areas, to come to some kind of consensus, whether it's local or national, about where these cut-off points should come. In fact, I think it is highly unlikely there *will* be a national policy in this area, but I know from experience that it is certainly a discussion that we are having locally with our cardiologists and it is also one that is very much alive in the tertiary centre that we use for these operations.

So what I'm saying, I suppose, is that at the moment we largely have professionals making their own decisions as they see them; but if we were to move to a more explicit policy, it would have to be on the basis of discussion and agreement between the professionals and other groups. It wouldn't work unless the doctors agreed to it. And although it's dangerous to generalize, I think there are some clinicians who are certainly interested in that kind of discussion because some of them, off the record and informally, would recognize that patients are being treated who perhaps do not stand much chance of getting better – but they have to be treated simply because they have been on the waiting list for 18 months or 12 months or whatever it is.

Emergencies pose a different kind of problem. In Britain we have a culture and a national health service which says that if you're ill and you need emergency treatment, you will be admitted to hospital and you will get the treatment you need. Indeed, successive governments have always put the access to emergency secondary services pretty near the top of their list of priorities. So I think that culturally it's very unlikely that any government, and therefore any health authority, would have the stomach to say to someone, well you're 84 and so we will try to repair your ruptured aneurysm, but if you had been 85, I'm afraid we would have had to let you bleed to death. I really don't see this as something that is likely to work in Britain. Informally, of course, I recognize that it goes on all the time, even as we are now sitting here. But what I am saying, I think, is that no government would want to become involved in decisions about who to treat in an emergency. There are no votes in that other than lost votes. It's simply not going to be a rewarding thing to do politically. It's too controversial for even the most bullish of governments to get into. No, it's in relation to elective treatments that a groundswell of opinion is growing within the professions that this is at least something they should be discussing. And I think there are signs that it is beginning to happen.

But if we are to go farther down this road, we will have to find ways of bringing the public on board. After all, we are making decisions about how public money is spent on the health care of the public. Health authorities are public institutions and they are charged with making these sorts of decisions; so yes, it is entirely appropriate that those who are paying for the services and those who are receiving them should have the opportunity to understand and be informed about the circumstances in which they will or will not receive treatment. It is part and parcel of the democratic society. There has been a lot of guidance from government about the proper role of the public in decision-making in the health service, but it's a very difficult area and not one where I profess any great insight. But what I would say is that it seems to me to be right in principle that the public should have the opportunity, if they wish, to be involved in decision-making.

There is an ethical dimension to this as well. When the health authority had to reach a decision on sub-fertility services, there was undoubtedly a role for members of the health authority to say, ethically, whether they thought the service should be provided only to people who were in a stable relationship. And the individual members of the health authority did just that: they said that they believed it was right to make this restriction. So yes, there is clearly an ethical dimension to these kinds of decisions. Where I have problems, at least in my own mind, is that what is right for one person may be wrong for someone else. In other words there are no absolute standards that we have the right to apply to everyone. There's clearly a great deal of subjectivity in all of our individual thinking about ethics, and health authority members are free to apply their own ethical views to whatever decisions they are making. That's not an unreasonable thing for them to do. They are on the health authority to make decisions, and the Secretary of State thinks they are the kind of people who should be making them.

Having said that, however, it does seem to me that health authorities are best advised to steer clear of issues about personal ethics and to make decisions about rationing on the basis of established evidence about what works and what doesn't work. Should we provide triple therapy for people with HIV and AIDS? Well, the first question – perhaps the only question – we should be asking is whether it works. Does it make people better? If the answer to that is yes, then it should be available and you can then set clinical criteria against which it will be prescribed. What we *shouldn't* do is to begin by asking whether it is ethical to provide triple therapy. We shouldn't say that because most people contract the HIV virus through things that we don't approve of, like intravenous drug use or homosexual contacts, then we won't make it available. That seems to me to be the wrong way of going about things. It should not be a primary consideration. Indeed, I don't think it should be a consideration at all. So the evidence that something works is much more important than whether a health authority thinks a particular behaviour is or is not ethically acceptable.

The district nurse's story

Rationing runs like a thread through our care, but in the community it seems to be hidden rationing. We always have an underlying feeling that we're struggling to match resources to needs, and we are always having to bear cost-effectiveness in the back of our minds when we're doing things. It's a general feeling that you're always trying to match resources – which aren't as good as they should be – to the needs of the population. A lot of it comes down to time: there always seem to be more things to do than you have time to do them. It's a very common thing running throughout our work. But it's not only time. It can also affect supplies and equipment.

For example, we have a continence policy in our district which involves the supply of pads for people who need them. About five years ago the Trust introduced a new eligibility policy for these products. Only three categories of patients are entitled to have them: those with very debilitating illnesses like multiple sclerosis and dementia, those who have had continence problems as a result of surgery, and those who reach the social services criteria of eligibility for continuing care. If patients need incontinence pads but they don't meet the criteria, all we can do is to give them information about where they can buy them. For example, if we had a little old lady whose rheumatoid arthritis was stopping her from getting to the toilet on time and she was often wet, she wouldn't qualify because she wouldn't have a debilitating illness. We would have to say to her, look, I'm sorry but you will have to go out and buy the pads yourself. If she couldn't afford them, she might end up with sore skin and a district nurse would then have to visit even more frequently to attend to her. We are in a fairly affluent area here and a lot of people can afford to buy the pads; but many can't, and it's definitely an example of rationing.

For some patients it's simply a matter of comfort and convenience, but for others it means a poor standard of care. In the past you used to be able to help them – you could often find some kind of evidence of dementia in their case-notes and then you could fit them into one of the approved categories. But now we have to fill in a special assessment form and send it to the continence service and they vet all our applications. They will throw them out if they don't think that we have met the criteria. You feel very bad about it because you're in the house, right at the bedside. Sometimes the relatives and carers take it out on you, often when it's a younger person caring for an older person and they're the ones who are having to do the washing and the caring. It's a dilemma isn't it? It's an ethical dilemma. When it was first introduced we put across our misgivings to the managers. We said it would be counter-productive of our time because we may end up treating more patients with pressure sores; but it was nevertheless imposed on us. The whole ethos is to be cost-effective within a fixed budget, so there we are. It's a repeating story. That's rationing for you.

Another example is the Marie Curie nursing service which is available to terminally ill patients in their own homes. The Marie Curie nurses usually work at night. We are responsible for the day care of patients who are dying, but when they become very ill and it's clear that they are going to die at home, the Marie Curie nurses will be in the house between 10.00 in the evening and 7.00 in the morning to do whatever is needed. But because the trust has only a limited budget for it, the service is rationed and we're only allowed to use the nurses for three nights a week. If we go to a fourth night, then a manager will ring us up and ask why we are doing it. Is it really warranted? And then we have to justify our position, but this is very difficult – you don't know exactly when a patient is going to die, and the Marie Curie nurse will be most needed right at the very end.

So what you tend to do is to book the Marie Curie nurse for the nights you think she will be needed, and worry about it later. I had a lady last year who had 14 nights altogether because her husband was very anxious and he needed somebody there. He couldn't really cope but he did want his wife to die at home. So I had to ring up the manager who deals with the Marie Curie service, and every three nights I had to justify the continuing booking to her in a telephone conversation. I felt I shouldn't have had to do that. The silly part of it is that provided you keep to the rule of three nights a week, nobody asks you any questions. I have another lady who has been dying for a year now, and she had Marie Curie set up last August for three nights a week because that was all I was allowed to give her. The family do the other four nights, though it isn't very easy for them because her children have all got busy jobs and they can't always be there with her. So we've kept the service going for her. She's had three nights of Marie Curie every week for almost a year now, and nobody has phoned me up! It's a standing joke! The budget must be going through the roof and I'm waiting for somebody to phone me up every week; but nobody ever does. It's ridiculous. And yet I had to fight to get 14 nights for the other lady and her anxious husband. It's not right, is it?

Leg ulcers are another example. When we ran a leg ulcer clinic we used a system of compression bandaging called four-layer bandaging. It was developed from research done at the Charing Cross Hospital, and we were encouraged by the Trust to use it because it was known to be effective. So we did. Then, after the clinic had been running for about a couple of years, my manager wanted to know why the budget for dressings was £1,000 higher than anywhere else; and of course the reason was that the four-layer bandaging doesn't come on prescription. We were ordering the bandages from our central stores, and this was quite costly

– about £8 a time – and it had to be done at least weekly. So my manager identified the bandaging as the blip in the dressing budget and he wanted me to change it to a single pressure bandage which was available on prescription and therefore came out of the GPs' budget.

We argued that although the single bandage was very effective in certain cases, patients who had exuding ulceration, for instance, needed the four layers to contain it. So we said that we would go on with that system because it was research-based and we weren't prepared to change. In fact the Trust had actually audited the care of leg ulcers across the district with very good results, so they couldn't very well then say that we were wrong. We're still using the more expensive bandages and our budget is still overspent; but fortunately the Trust is still paying. It's an example of how on the one hand they want you to follow good research-based practice, but when you actually spend the money you come up against resistance.

I know more about leg ulcers than most district nurses because I've actually been running a leg ulcer clinic, and I feel that I'm quite good at stating my case; so the managers haven't been able to stop me ordering the bandages in the usual way. The ulcers in my patients are healing, and I have the evidence to prove it. So if the managers ask me why I should have the bandages when district nurses elsewhere are managing without them, we can say it's because our patients are doing better than theirs. But I do think that other district nurses are finding that the policy is quite rigid and is very rigorously vetted. Perhaps their managers have put more pressure on them, or maybe they haven't been so assertive. I do see it as an ethical problem because our patients are getting a better service than elsewhere in the district. But at least we have tried to get other places to do what we are doing.

Now that we have nurse prescribing, the GPs are also wanting to know what we're doing. Take catheters. Before, if we needed a catheter, we would just ask a GP for whichever catheter was right for that patient; but now, if there are two or three manufacturers making the same type and one is slightly cheaper than the others, we will go for the cheaper one. You've always got at the back of your mind that at the end of the year the GPs are going to look at our figures, and if we're prescribing large volumes of something that is expensive, they may say they're going to put a limit on our budget. It all comes down to how the GPs use their prescribing budget. Take patients with exuding wounds or ulcers who are losing a lot of protein. There are supplementary drinks that GPs can prescribe – which we can't – which are very beneficial for the nutrition of elderly patients in getting their wounds to heal; but they are expensive. If the doctors won't prescribe the drinks, there's nothing we can do. It is a real issue: patients may need three drinks a day, and that's 21 drinks a week and it's a lot of money.

But it's not only money: time is also a problem. There's never enough time to do everything you want to, and so you have to learn how to prioritize your work. It's something that you do on the hoof, really. You do it as you go along – intuitively. You may have somebody at the end of your list who is not particularly desperate for that day, and you end up having to phone them and apologize and say I'm ever so sorry, I've had a very busy day. Most people are very accommodating, but if their dressing is due that day, then you haven't really got any choice but to work overtime. That then encroaches on your personal time, so you try to take it back from the next day's or week's work – but that's not always possible. You can quite easily accumulate whole days of overtime in a short space, and if you then take a day back, that puts pressure on the other members of staff. It's a vicious cycle. But always you have to give the patients the time they need. So yes, you are forever juggling with time. You have to decide which patients need you most.

I suppose in a lot of our work we are a buffer between our patients and our managers, and it's wrong in my view that we should be in that position. Perhaps the way our work is funded should be more individualized. Perhaps we should even have our own budgets, because we know what our patients need and we would then be able to spend the money to get the best results. At the moment, everything is so far away and this makes it more difficult to explain to patients that they can't have this or they can't do that because of a budget that's been fixed by managers who know nothing about them at all. But if you actually knew the limits of your own budget, you could say, I'm ever so sorry, but I've also got to look after another patient who is dying or who needs a lot of care. You would have a bit more authority to make these judgments. At the moment, though, it can be difficult. You can't actually tell patients who are dying that they can't have a Marie Curie nurse. So I'll say to them that they can have a nurse if they really need one, and it's then my responsibility to fix it with my manager.

Sometimes I have to say well, that's the policy of the Trust and if you really feel very strongly about it then I can put you in touch with a manager and you can talk to him about it. It becomes really difficult when you have carried out an assessment on a patient and you then can't do anything for them because of budgetary limitations. It can be quite traumatic. For instance, a lot of the equipment that allows us to nurse patients at home is limited – rationed if you like. Equipment for bathing used to be available to everybody as long as we assessed them and found they were having difficulty getting in and out of the bath. But then we were told that we would only be able to provide it for patients who had had surgery, like hip replacements or knee replacements, or who were terminally ill. So we have to say to patients who don't come into either category that we recommend they should get a bath seat, but they will have to buy it themselves. And if they don't buy the seat, there is a possibility that they may slip or fall in the bath and hurt themselves.

We have a policy for joint assessment and eligibility between ourselves and social services. If you're nursing a patient at home who requires a package of both health and social care, there's an eligibility criteria document which tells you whether a patient's needs are mostly health or mostly social. A decision is then made between the care manager and the district nurse about the package of care that will be supplied. If it's a social service carer, the patient may have to pay a fee, but if it's a nurse, the patients pay nothing. This can create problems for us, because if you have a patient whose needs are mostly health, that's going to put an awful lot of demands on the district nursing service. Often we simply don't have the personnel to deliver the package. But as soon as a social services carer goes in, there may be a cost element to the patient; so there may be pressure to make more use of the district nurses because the patient won't have to pay.

I've got no doubt that patients should be cared for in the community as far as they possibly can be, and they should be kept out of hospital. But the way the health authority and social services have developed the joint eligibility criteria has made it quite difficult for district nurses to deliver the care that the patient needs. If you are doing a joint assessment on a patient with a care manager and you say that you haven't enough nurses to deliver the package properly, the care manager will say well, we can't do any more than half the visits because we're over our budget already. So we're fighting our corner and they're fighting theirs and the patients are in the middle. We can agree on what they need, but that's the easy bit. The difficulty comes over who is actually going to deliver the care. If you don't think things are right you always have recourse to your own manager, and then you can argue with social services, and then if necessary you can go to the next level.

I had one patient whose case we argued all the way through because it was a particularly difficult situation. He had motor neurone disease and he couldn't move himself at all. The only way he could communicate was by laughing or moving his face. He had a catheter and a tube to enable him to feed, and because of all these things his skin was vulnerable to pressure. He was on a special bed. According to the eligibility criteria he was a very dependent patient whose needs were mainly health, and we were told that we had to do most of the care. But in fact he was actually very stable and really only needed what I would call social care – social bathing, dressing, turning, that kind of thing. You don't necessarily need a nurse to do that. He'd also got a very supportive family who wanted to be involved in his care and were very willing to do things like feeding him through the tube. So we argued that to put in nursing care in a double-handed visit three times a day would have been just too much, and we agreed in the end that we would provide half the package of care. We would supply the special mattress, monitor his pressure areas, give advice on moving and handling him, keep an eye on his catheter and tube, and support the family. We said that if social services would do the two morning visits and the evening one, we would meet up with one of the carers and do the lunchtime visit. So you have to be very flexible to achieve a package of care that is acceptable to the family, to the nursing service and to social services and that also meets all the budgets and criteria. Thankfully there aren't many patients out there like that, probably only about half a dozen of them on my case load, but it's quite a difficult business working your way through the criteria.

One of the problems with staffing is the lack of any backup, particularly for sick leave or holidays. We don't get any extra nurses and we just have to stretch ourselves further. It's not like a hospital ward where you have 32 beds and when they're full that's it. In a community, you could have 10 patients on your case load or 100 patients. You just have to stretch to accommodate them, and if people are off sick or on holiday there's no extra help. We do have a system of flexi-bank staff but it can be very difficult to get hold of them, particularly during school holidays. In any case, they're not trained in the same way that we are and they may never have worked in the community. So even if you have the benefit of a flexi-bank nurse, she may never have been to your town before and she may only have done a few hours in the community. If you're very busy, you simply haven't got the time to sit down and tell her what to do on that day. You just have to give her a list of patients and send her off; and often you find that the following day you may pick up problems because perhaps the dressing hasn't been done in quite the right way.

The neurologist's story

The first thing that I would say about rationing is that to quite a large extent neurologists have been able to pick and choose what they will do, and this is why there is a widespread perception that neurology is rationed very tightly. The demand for services connected with the nervous system is very large, and unlike many other countries, there are relatively few neurologists in the NHS – only about 200 – mostly dealing with rare diseases. This results in rationing, because although there has been a small increase in the number of neurologists, it has simply not been possible to meet the demand that has been created for their services. Although it is a small specialty, there are substantial numbers of people now who want to see a neurologist.

Control of this demand is done partly by resisting the pressure to become too involved in district general hospitals. There has been something of a movement of neurologists into the districts, but most neurologists have retained a regional base. They've done this partly for good medical reasons but partly as a conscious way of rationing their services. If you're not easily available locally you can't be easily consulted. And then, of course, the waiting list imposes a certain structure on how many patients one can see and what one does. No initiative that I ever encountered has brought a neurological waiting list down for more than a short period of time, because all that happens is that people who have been seeing a general physician or a geriatrician – or who haven't been referred at all – suddenly turn up to fill the holes in the list. In this hospital there are six clinics in neurology, which represent about 12 sessions if you take into account the administrative time; but we'd need something in the region of 50 to 60 sessions a week if we were to see every single problem affecting the nervous system that is referred to the hospital out-patient's departments.

The main filter, of course, is the GP. He's the gatekeeper. He determines what gets sent to the neurologist and what goes elsewhere. So the GP may say to himself, I recognize that this is a neurological problem, but I think it could be handled more quickly by sending the patient to an ophthalmologist or a general surgeon or whatever. You can get paradoxical things happening because of this. For instance, one of the real medical emergencies to do with stroke is a transient ischaemic attack, which is basically a warning that a stroke may be impending. However, I see very few of these patients although I have a stated interest in the organization of cerebro-vascular services, because of the length of my waiting list and because I have been discouraged for financial reasons from setting up a service to deal with them.

The waiting lists are managed by prioritizing the patients, usually on the basis of the GP's referral letter. Although neurology has a reputation of being very cerebral, in many cases it has more to do with pattern recognition. It's triage. Just that. You schedule patients' appointments as 'urgent', 'soon' or 'routine'. If a patient gets a 'routine' appointment, then a fairly complex set of dynamics may develop between the GP, the patient and the neurologist. The classical example of this is possible multiple sclerosis, where the GP says that he doesn't think the patient has got MS but is not absolutely sure. So you look at the symptoms in the letter and you think that if the probability of MS is very low, there is no medical justification for prioritizing the patient. But the patient may have convinced himself that he *has* got MS, and he will then badger the GP who in turn will badger me. It's arguable that there might then be a social justification for moving the patient up the list, but one is then apportioning limited resources both on the basis of medical needs and the patient's wishes, which are not necessarily identical.

Triage is not foolproof. Sometimes I get it wrong because I misinterpret the letter. When this happens the GP will usually say, look, I'm not happy about this, the patient has signs and symptoms that are evolving and changing. And then the patient can be seen sooner. So there is always a certain amount of interplay, although because of this the system is open to abuse. Some patients and GPs know that the more they press the better are their chances of being seen sooner rather than later.

Sometimes there is actually a positive value in patients being delayed before coming to see me. Take the case of patients with early dementia. In my experience, investigation, though very expensive, adds little to the clinical impression and does not help medical management. However, it is very difficult not to respond to the uncertainty and worry of patients and relatives by undertaking the tests they want, even though I feel these will help far less diagnostically than the passage of time. The money spent on these tests would be much better directed towards improving care for patients later on.

Another example is someone who has a possible epileptic fit for the first time. The chance of this occurring in a lifetime is about one in 30, and the overall chance of this turning into epilepsy, with a recurring liability to seizures, is about 20 per cent. Logically, one way to deal with a first attack is to see the patient, decide whether it's a fit or not, and then wait to see what happens. If the patient really does have epilepsy, then there's a reasonably good chance of a second fit occurring within three months; so if I delay the process by 12 weeks, I'm likely to be diagnostically more accurate. But of course this doesn't happen in private medicine, because as soon as somebody has a fit they come and see me and then I'm forced to act. I can't just say look, you shouldn't be seeing me yet, let's just wait and see what happens. I'm forced to be proactive, not necessarily because it is medically good but to satisfy the desires of the patient who's paying me.

Private medicine also forms a type of rationing. For instance, if the GP does not feel there is a medical justification for the patient being seen urgently but the patient does, then it's open to them to ask for a private consultation. Where it is a matter of reassurance, I don't feel at all bad about it. The patients have paid for their peace of mind, and there's nothing wrong with that. Where I do feel bad – very bad, sometimes – is where there is a real problem that I have failed to pick up at the beginning when the patient is first referred. It doesn't happen very often, but when it does, it's upsetting. You've labelled a patient as 'routine' and you wouldn't normally see them for quite some time; but then they pay to see you privately and you realize that you got it wrong. The patient really does have MS or whatever. Although they're embarrassing, these cases are instructive because they provide a check of sorts on how well the system is working.

I think there is another unspoken use of long waiting lists, though it is not acknowledged, and this concerns the length of time that certain groups of people have to wait. These groups, the 'heart-sink' patients, the multiple re-attenders, often finish up in the vague area of the waiting list where clinical responsibility for them can be diffused. To begin with it's the GP who is responsible, but as soon as you put them on the 'routine' list the GP can say to them, 'I'm very sorry, there's nothing I can do because you're waiting to see the neurologist. I'm sorry if you have to wait six or nine months, but that's because you're going to see a very important person'. It happens less often here than it used to when I worked elsewhere, but it still exists.

The medical risk of long waiting lists, of course, is that potentially serious conditions could be missed while patients are waiting. Before easy access to CT scans, I reckoned I was delaying the diagnosis of perhaps one brain tumour a year by having a long waiting list, and from time to time it still happens that I gravely misread the referral letter. On other occasions the referral letter suggests that there are no grounds for treating the case as urgent but in fact the patient is brewing up something which they're presenting in a different way. I'm not too worried when this happens, given the resources that are available to us, and we deal with it by maintaining the potential for rapid access by the GP. But it is a situation that new consultants, in particular, always fear. They look at their mounting waiting lists and they think goodness, there must be some sick people here who haven't been picked up.

Once the patient actually gets to see me, I'm conscious the whole time that I am using resources for which there is competition. I try to give patients the time that they need and I frequently run into trouble by overrunning clinic times; but that's not the real rationing issue for me. It's not time. It's really to do with three things: sophisticated tests, admission to the neurosciences unit, and whether the available treatment can be afforded.

Take the tests. I always try to under-investigate rather than over-investigate patients, particularly if it involves the use of sophisticated scanning such as MRI. I'm conscious of two things. One is that these investigations are expensive and they are only available in limited amounts; and if I don't myself indulge in good housekeeping, then I can hardly take a strong line with others who seem to be over-using the system. The other is that, if you are really confident about what you are doing, you don't need to order a whole series of tests. I'm very aware, however, that many of my investigations are for medico-legal reasons, and this is a constant source of concern because I think it is clinically and financially wrong. On the other hand, I do need to be able to justify what I am doing because I always have at the back of my mind that my actions may be scrutinized by lawyers.

The second area of rationing occurs over admissions to the neurosciences unit. In our region there used to be five neurologists covering a region of more than three million people with access to 40 beds. Now there are 20 neurologists for the same area with access to 32 beds. So this means that it is becoming increasingly difficult for neurologists to get their patients into hospital and many fewer patients are now admitted. Of course, not so many patients need admission now, but certainly some patients are not getting into hospital who would be managed better if they were admitted. If I can get a patient into hospital and quickly sorted out, then they need fewer subsequent appointments, as all the necessary tests can be done at the same time. But if they're seen in out-patients, then it drags on and takes up a lot more time.

The third question is whether the available treatment can be afforded. A good example is the treatment of Parkinson's disease. This is a condition for which new drugs are being brought out all the time such as Beta Interferon, which I think is one of the best paradigms for talking about the rationing of treatment. In this area there are about 570 patients with multiple sclerosis. It used to be untreatable, but really good evidence has emerged over the last four years that under certain circumstances significant alterations to the natural history can be made by giving Beta Interferon. During the three years of the first North American trial, the number of relapses dropped by 30 per cent and the number of severe relapses dropped by 50 per cent. The changes on the MRI were quite astonishing. For somebody with relapsing MS there is now a drug which will reduce the rate of deterioration.

But it comes at a cost. Ten thousand pounds per person per year, to be precise, and we have estimated that about 220 of the 570 MS patients in this area would be eligible for Beta Interferon on an open-ended commitment. The consequence of this would be a bill of about £2,200,000 per year for the health authority – which they feel they cannot afford. So we had to decide upon a mechanism for rationing the drug. Initially we did it by working in close co-operation with the MS societies, and we were helped by their responsible attitude which was 'let's hold back for a moment, let's be careful, there are side effects and we don't know what will happen in the long term'.

But as one would expect, the use of Beta Interferon began to creep up, and new evidence began to emerge about its benefits for a wider group of patients with MS. This became even more alarming in resource terms for the health authority, so the local neurologists had a meeting with them as we were unwilling for them to impose guidelines and protocols on us. We didn't think it was right that the health authority should decide who could and couldn't have the drug. Instead, we argued successfully for the devolution of a budget for which *we* would be responsible. So now it is expected that the neurologists will meet at various times during the year to review the patients whom we think are suitable for the drug. In fact the devolved budget covers only about a quarter of the people who should theoretically be eligible, but it seemed better for us to ration ourselves than to have it done for us by the health authority. In my experience the provider/commissioner split is divisive and unhelpful, and it seemed much better that we took the responsibility for what we could and couldn't do. There are many other examples of drug rationing. In this district Riluzole, the only proven drug for the treatment of motor neurone disease, cannot be given routinely because it is felt that the evidence does not justify the cost.

There are many other limitations in treatment, both with new drugs and with nursing and therapy, that can be offered to neurological patients, particularly those with chronic diseases. Although it is fair to say that much of this rationing comes from insufficient funding, it would not be fair to put all the blame on this. Part comes from a genuine shortage of nursing and paramedical resources, which is a demographic problem as well as one of poor pay. And the other, which I think is far more difficult to deal with, is that expectations of the health service will always run ahead of what it can actually provide; and I think that rationing will remain an inevitable part of any health service because of this.

The nursing manager's story

When we're thinking about rationing, we have to distinguish between two major types of resource inadequacies. One is human resources and the other is equipment. In terms of human resources, every ward or department has an agreed establishment which, for one reason or another, may not be adequate. The number of emergency admissions may have risen, or the bed occupancy levels may have increased, or the patients may be sicker or older or more dependent. A ward may always have had a low establishment or it may have a reasonable establishment but cannot recruit enough people to fill the posts. Specialist areas such as renal medicine and neonatal intensive care, for example, have immense difficulties in recruiting highly specialist nurses. So that's one issue: staffing. The other issue is the lack of equipment or the generally high level of demand that's made upon it. Patients are queuing up to come into the wards, so nurses often have to work at quite a fast pace and it doesn't let up. So one way or another, yes, the ultimate result is that there is a perceived and very often real impact on patient care.

Now, you ask me what nurses do about it. The first thing that nurses always have on their mind is their accountability to their patients, and that's based on their code of conduct. One of the clauses in the code clearly requires a qualified nurse to take action if she sees that a situation is detrimental to the well-being of her patient. So if you take the issue of the lack of staff, there's very often a number of things that can be done. For example, we have a flexi-bank service and we could try to get somebody in who could work a more flexible rota. Or we may borrow from other wards or make adjustments in one way or another. The important thing is that it is brought to the attention of the managers so that they can think about contingency plans. It may just be a matter of covering a single shift, but it might be a more prolonged period where staffing has been consistently at a level where care is compromised or may even be unsafe. So there are remedial actions that can be taken, but they are only going to work up to a point. Sometimes, and I have seen it happen, we have to take measures like closing beds or even closing a ward and moving our resources into another area. I would say that much of the time nowadays we are working right up to the line and sometimes beyond it in terms of managing demands against our resources. It's a major headache.

In terms of patient care, this can mean two things. First, we end up with a stressed workforce. Morale dips, sickness levels go up, people are working longer hours, and generally they are frustrated and emotional. When you've got a nursing workforce that is stressed and very pushed, you cannot expect it to give a consistently good standard of care. It's just not possible. So secondly, what they have to do is to prioritize their activities so that they do what is necessary to maintain the basic level of safety. When the demands on them are such that they cannot meet all their patients' needs, they will have to prioritize their work. Basically, the demands come from two sources. One is our elective admissions, and while we have the waiting list initiative there is a continual pressure on us not to cancel planned admissions. But there are also demands for emergency admissions which are enormous at times. One would expect it to peak in the winter months and then drop down in the summer, but this year we have had a consistently enormous demand on our emergency admissions right the way through the year. We haven't had the respite that we would expect to allow us to increase our elective activity. There are some exceptions. Paediatrics tend to be much busier in the winter because of all the children with respiratory diseases, so at the moment it is quite quiet. But I would say that at least one part of the hospital is really struggling at any particular time.

And these are not just isolated occurrences. I've noticed throughout my nursing career that we expect more and more from our nursing staff. It's a much more common phenomenon than I would wish and it's not consistent with an expectation of a good standard of care all the time. We are finding an increasing number of errors, such as drug errors. When staff are tired and stressed, they can't be expected to do complex calculations about drug doses and that sort of thing. And the patients that we have nowadays are mostly very ill and dependent. These days, if you can get out of bed and put your slippers on, then you're discharged. So both the pace and the intensity of work on the ward are so much quicker, and there may well be times when safety could be called into question. When patients first come into the hospital they are at risk from a number of potential problems. We should be doing risk assessments and preventing those problems from happening in the first place by a series of actions. But if the assessments are not carried out and the actions are not put into place, then patients may, for example, get pressure sores because they have not had the level of attention that they need. I would say that that's a safety issue: something is happening to them that is deleterious to their health that wouldn't have happened if they had had the proper input of care.

There are a number of indicators we can use to pick this up. One of them is simply to look at the experiences that patients have of their stay in hospital, and we do that. But we have to bear in mind that patients usually get better in spite of any limitations in their care. They get the treatment they need, safely, and that's it. What they may not get is the psychological support they need, or the information they need, or the holding of the hand in the small hours when they're feeling desperate. They may not get all of that. They won't die as a result, but it will colour their experience of being in hospital. The amount of caring in its truest sense will to a large extent depend upon the availability of the resources to give it.

I could give you lots of examples. When the meal trolley arrives on the ward, we should be giving out the meals straight away. If you don't serve them within a certain period of time you shouldn't be serving them at all. Not only that, patients should have their meals at an appropriate temperature, otherwise it puts them off eating. It's better for them to have a good balanced meal rather than dietary supplements later on because their meal has got cold and we have had to take it away.

Drug rounds are another example. They must take place at the appropriate times because the drugs must be correctly spaced. But a nurse may be constantly interrupted when she is doing a drug round, and it doesn't help her concentration when she's got complex drug calculations to make. Nowadays we give a lot of intravenous drugs. On a surgical ward you may find up to 14 sets of intravenous drugs being administered. That is very time-consuming. So the only way we can cope is by delegating basic care – things like hygiene and toileting – to unqualified staff. So this is another area that does have an impact on patient care. Obviously an unqualified nurse works under the supervision of a trained nurse, but the point is that because she is not trained herself, it affects the quality of care we can give our patients. Very often nowadays the trained nurse is tied up with running the ward, doing the drug rounds, dealing with enquiries and so on, and the actual basic care is being given by care assistants.

Of course, skill mix and grade mix have always been with us. On any ward there will be, maybe, 60 or 70 per cent of trained nurses and 30 or 40 per cent untrained. It will vary according to the type of ward. The less technology there is on a ward, the more likely there is to be a higher untrained workforce. I think one of the greatest losses is that we used to have student nurses on the wards throughout their three-year programme, and we certainly had a mix on any ward of 1st, 2nd and 3rd year students. By the time they came to the 2nd or 3rd years they were actually very valuable members of the team. That has now finished, and all we have is some flitting in and out of the wards during their programme; and because they've had so little exposure to working in an acute setting, they have a lot to learn and cannot offer much themselves. That is a great loss. Of course, you could argue that they were used and abused, but now we use and abuse health care assistants instead.

Bed management is another thing that has created immense pressures and tensions within the hospital. We can go from a situation where we may have about 30 beds in the evening and we are well set for taking in emergencies during the night to one in which we've only one or two available beds. When that happens we have to make the consultants very aware that the bed situation is extremely tight and that if possible they should increase their discharges. So patients could be going home as soon as they can get their slippers on. At the same time we have to bear in mind our waiting lists and we have to categorize them. For example, there may be patients with cancer who have to be admitted fairly quickly. But we mustn't forget about patients who have been on the waiting list for a long time and we also have to think about those who are vocal. Patients sometimes ring in to find out whether there's a bed available, and they get very vocal and angry because they feel their case is as important as anybody else's – which of course it is, for them. We have to balance all of this against the need to accommodate emergency admissions and we have to decide what we are going to do if we can't admit all the emergencies that occur.

Sometimes we have to close the hospital to new admissions, though we do our very best to keep it open. We have a bed management policy and there are some beds, in gynaecology or surgery for example, that are withdrawn from ring-fenced use when we are moving into a bed crisis. We put them into the general bed pool because we simply have to accommodate patients who are very sick and need to be admitted. Sometimes we have to use extra areas which aren't supposed to have in-patients. I've known patients to be accommodated in endoscopy for example, which is only an out-patient service but there are a few beds there. The bottom line is whether it is safe. Are there enough nurses in that area to meet the core needs of the patients who are being accommodated there? Another thing we can do is to move patients from high-risk beds if they have been in hospital for three or four days and are due to go home. The patients don't like that. They're settled and they've got to know the nurses in their ward and they don't want to move. Sometimes a patient will be moved a number of times during his in-patient stay, which is not good for continuity of care but there is nothing else that we can do. We find ourselves frequently between a rock and a hard place. You just don't know what to do for the best. It does sometimes pit manager against manager. 'You can't use my beds . . .' That's the sort of conversation that goes on and it is very difficult.

Another problem is that we may, overnight, have to admit patients and accommodate them in an area that is just for electives such as day surgery, and then the day surgery nurses turn up in the morning only to find patients in the beds designated for their 7 a.m. admissions. It really is very difficult. We have now developed a discharge lounge so that patients can be moved out of their beds first thing in the morning on their day of discharge and sit in a lounge chair until their drugs are ready and their relatives can collect them. There are all sorts of strategies we have to try. It's no different to any other hospital. I often go to other hospitals and they have exactly the same experiences.

Clearly decisions about the clinical management of patients have to be led by the clinicians, but I would stress that it should be in consultation with the patients and their relatives and it must take account of the patients' own wishes. Of course, this immediately raises ethical issues. Are we going to do the greatest good for the greatest number, or are we going to think about the individual? My observation is that doctors have always been in a dilemma about this because what they actually think about when they are with a patient is what is right for that particular patient. You can't criticize them for this because it's what they're trained to do. But nowadays, with the NHS reforms, there's greater and greater pressure for doctors to have a keen eye on the budget, particularly if they are clinical directors.

The bottom line is the budget. There's a limited pocket of money and we can't ignore the fact. So in terms of decisions that have to be taken in life-threatening situations, I would say that good practice would require the doctors to take proper account of the wishes of the patient and his relatives and also to involve other professionals – nurses, physiotherapists, and other disciplines as necessary. If it's a dire emergency, then the clinicians will do all they can to save the patient, but they will have to decide when the point is reached at which the patient's situation has become irretrievable. And uncomfortable decisions are also having to be made about what treatment a patient might *not* have. Some of the cancer drugs such as Taxol are obvious examples of this. Different health authorities have different views about these very expensive treatments, and you can have a situation where people in one street can benefit from an expensive drug while those in the next street can't. So those types of difficult decisions are certainly being made about major treatments.

One thing that we haven't touched on yet is the whole question of waste in the NHS and the inappropriateness of treatments such as dilatation and curettage and grommets, which have been called into question. My own view is that we have to respect the clinical judgment of the doctors in cases like these. That is paramount. After all, they are the experts at whatever speciality they're in. It's fine to have guidelines or protocols or whatever, but there must always be the possibility of deviating from them; and that's what clinical judgment is all about. But nevertheless, I would say that there is waste in the NHS, particularly at a systems level. There are always ways to improve a system, even though it may require an initial investment of resources to find out what they are. Look at those hospitals which have gone into process re-engineering and integrated care pathways. But if you take the Leicester Royal Infirmary, which is being held up as an excellent example of process re-engineering, it required a big investment in the first place.

Nurses are also moving into areas that have traditionally been the territory of the doctors. We're seeing the advent of more and more specialist nurses with higher levels of knowledge and expertise, often in quite narrow areas. Nowadays these specialist nurses and nurse practitioners can very often carry out clinical tasks as well as, or often better than, the doctors, and this allows the doctors to use their time more effectively. In this hospital, for example, we've identified about 100 patients a week in clinical oncology who are currently seen by consultants because they're on radiotherapy treatment; but we are gradually moving to a situation in which they are being seen by the clinical nurse practitioner in the oncology department. Now that's a very good move, and I would certainly support it; but when we identified other specialist nursing posts that could be of equal value in improving the quality of care to patients and making clinicians more effective, our purchasers didn't want to know about it. I've been in dialogue with them for a couple of years now about epilepsy nurse specialists who could have a real impact on the quality of care for patients with epilepsy. But we can't get them funded. And so I have to write to pharmaceutical companies to see if we can get sponsorship any other way. Only last week I was interviewing for a specialist nurse in vascular work, and we've had to fund it through a private route. It's not ideal, but she will make an enormous impact on patients with vascular disease. So it's a nettle that I feel we need to grasp to improve the care of patients, particularly those with chronic diseases, and to make our clinicians more effective with their time. But we can't get the funding for it. It's immensely frustrating.

The public health physician's story

At one point in my career I worked overseas, somewhere with real resource problems. I came back from six months in a Russian winter where the temperature never got above $-22°$ and patients discharged themselves from hospital because the conditions were so bad they would rather be homeless on the streets. When I got back, everyone started complaining to me about the resource problems in the NHS, and I thought, you lot don't know you're born. Part of what I was doing in Russia was trying to persuade the doctors that they could no longer afford to do it like that. I was having to say to them look, you've only got this much money and if you carry on treating people the way you are, you are really only treating one person with maybe a 99 per cent chance of cure. But if you treat much less expensively with an 80 per cent chance of cure, then you'll be able to treat all of your patients. You'll have to start thinking about those sorts of choices.

That set me thinking about rationing in a very explicit way. A lot of people aren't prepared to take on board the fact that we must explicitly trade off the cost of treating one patient really well against the benefit of treating many more patients less well. I think people don't like to face up to it. If you've got 100 patients and you could treat all of them at an 80 per cent chance of cure, then you've got 80 cured patients. But if you could treat one of them at 99 per cent chance of cure, then you're likely to have cured only one patient at the end. So if it's 80 people versus one person, I'm voting for the 80. Otherwise you've also got 99 people who you don't treat at all. That doesn't seem right. Of course, these kinds of choices are not as explicit here as they were in Russia. The situation there is a lot more extreme. But the principle is just the same.

When I came to work at this authority, almost the first thing I had to do was to confront the authority's budget deficit. We decided that we obviously had to make some cuts with that kind of deficit, so we got a group of surgeons together to develop a contract restrictions policy. It was an extreme situation for them, but they were willing to consider what we were proposing. Initially we thought, let's try and use the QALY approach to see if some surgical activities are better value for money than others, but eventually we decided that it wasn't going to work. Why? Because we had to get our financial framework sorted out within a very short space of time and we didn't have enough time to tackle all the technical problems. If you are going to look at all the possible conditions that people might have, they would cover a huge number of procedures in general surgery. So we had to ask ourselves how we could make a balanced choice between them. Should we just do it on pain and discomfort? If so, how would we know that people weren't cheating the system? Then other ideas about the value of individuals began to impinge. Suppose you had a large family or you were a carer – should that mean you got extra points? There were so many imponderables that we gave up, partly for technical reasons but also for the practical reason that we had to get the financial framework sorted out.

So our approach to the list of contract restrictions was simply to ask ourselves what was acceptable – not a systematic way at all. The restrictions include cosmetic surgery, the reversal of sterilization and vasectomy, varicose veins unless they're very severe, and complementary therapies. In some cases we don't buy them at all; in others we buy them in restricted volume. For example, you can only have cosmetic surgery in exceptional individual circumstances. So if you've got a lump or a bump that's not causing you a functional problem and it's not on your face, then you will only have it removed in exceptional circumstances. Your GP or consultant must write to us here, and your case will then be considered by the Committee for Extra-Contractual Referrals (ECRs). But if you've got a lump that is disfiguring your face, then you will go through on the criteria alone and your case won't have to come to the ECR Committee at all. And if you've got a lump on your bottom so that you can't sit down, then it is a functional problem and it will also go through on the criteria.

As I said, the choices were made in a very pragmatic way – *ad hoc*, almost. Well, that's a polite way of describing it. What really happened was that we took advice from the clinicians as to what could work, but we made it clear that the buck stops with us at the health authority. We produce leaflets to tell the public what we are doing and what people can and cannot have done for them. It actually works really quite well; but if we have to go through the exercise again, I would involve the GPs and the CHC [Community Health Council] at a much earlier stage. Because we were pressed for time, we involved the surgeons a lot and only later went out to the GPs and the CHC. Almost all of the GPs were on board, and it helped that the fund-holders said that they were going along with the policy. Of course, we had a let-out clause under the exceptional individual circumstances, but in fact it hasn't been used that much. The ECR Committee now meets every month and it's getting fewer and fewer referrals – usually only one or two at each meeting.

Of course, you could argue that the policy has been acceptable to the professions and the public precisely because there aren't too many exclusions on the list. And it also helps that although I talk a lot to the press about it, they don't usually ask me the difficult questions. I take the view that if they ask me, I'll tell them where the gaps are, because we are arguing the case mainly on effectiveness grounds. If you read the literature on the randomized control trials of homeopathy, you'll find that it's not effective. I'm quite happy to defend that. It's different with something like cosmetic surgery, which is usually a very effective treatment. But it wasn't a problem for us to put that on the list: we just took the view that we couldn't afford it. We had savings to make, and in that situation cosmetic surgery is obviously less important than hip replacements.

In fact the exclusions have allowed us to save only a proportion of our target, but what they have done is to get people talking about explicit rationing, and I would say that this is the major plus point. The surgeons realized that we were prepared to stand up and tell people that we couldn't buy everything, and this forced them to start thinking about rationing in much more explicit ways than they had done previously.

This enabled us to talk to them about the cuts that we were planning to make to their elective surgery budgets, and we agreed a whole bundle of percentage reductions from different budgets. We tried to do it on a logical basis, but we didn't have very much of the information we needed. So we had to say well, we know we're under-purchasing major orthopaedic procedures because our hip replacement rates are really low, so we won't cut that; but we will cut general surgery, for example, or urology, because we know we can make some savings there.

So different percentages were agreed, and then there was a lot of *ad hoc* negotiating around them. The surgeons were really rather unhappy with us in public health and with some of the people in commissioning, but we had to say well, this is the best we can do about making sensible cuts. Some of this was hidden rationing, and most people really didn't know what was happening. I'm not happy about this. Since then we've tried to extend the exercise to medicine, but it's largely been unsuccessful. I think the reason is that we didn't have the pressure on the deficit. We specifically said that we were going to focus on respiratory disease, diabetes, gastro-intestinal disorders and other similar conditions. But the physicians have been talking largely about reorganizing services within their budgets rather than cutting them back. Unless there's a huge external pressure on people, they are not interested in rationalizing their work.

Even with clinical governance and primary care groups coming in, I think there's still a big gap around clinical autonomy. Health authorities are going to have to get involved in completely different ways now. Take, for example, follow-up cystoscopies for a bladder condition. It's entirely appropriate that people should be followed up with repeat cystoscopies, but this could be done on a much more evidence-based schedule. Some places *have* sorted themselves out a bit. Some models show that lots of places could cut about 15 per cent of their cystoscopy follow-ups. I did some work to calculate the number of misdiagnoses they might theoretically make by doing fewer cystoscopies, and I said to them, how do you feel about that – maybe that's a trade-off you might want to make? But it's been patchy.

Part of the problem is that not all of the clinicians are in control of their own budgets, and they are afraid that if they do save money by reducing their follow-up cystoscopies, they won't see any of the savings next year. So they say: what's the point of us doing that because we just lose it out of our budget. And then we'll do less with our time and we'll have less training. And I say, I agree with you, but if you don't accept the policy, others – and maybe you also – will lose out. For instance, one surgeon wasn't in the least interested in the contract restriction policy. It was a very clear-cut example. His unit had reduced its surgical activity by only a fraction of the others, and this was really inequitable. Some GPs said – not altogether jokingly – well, I'll refer all my veins to his unit, because they don't agree with the policy. That's not fair. And my biggest that's-not-fair gripe is the opportunity cost of it all, because if we spend the money on one unit that's doing too much, we can't spend it on something else. Some people don't seem to have worked it out that money is not elastic.

Drugs are another difficult issue. Viagra is going to be very expensive. Some GPs have calculated that it could take up to 20 per cent of their budgets. But that one hasn't really hit us yet. Beta Interferon is a really interesting one. I handled that one when I was working for a certain health authority and I thought we did it very well. The policy was that the drug would not be prescribed unless very strict criteria had been met, and everyone had signed up to it – all the local MS societies, all the local neurologists, some of the neighbouring districts' neurologists, and Uncle Tom Cobbleigh and all. Here, no-one seems quite to realize that if you overspend on one budget you have to take it out of somebody else's.

There's no really systematic way of making these kinds of decisions. It's done, quite frankly, in *ad hoc* ways. In the case of Aricept, we said to start with that it could be prescribed in exceptional individual circumstances. When we got a case through to the ECR Committee, we needed to know what would be regarded as exceptional circumstances. So we went back to the Prescribing Committee and said to them that they had to tell us what they regarded as an exceptional individual circumstance because we didn't know. Finally it was agreed – in fact at the last meeting of the Prescribing Committee – that they would take it on board. So now whenever a new drug appears, they will decide whether or not it is to be generally available, and if not, the particular circumstances under which it could be prescribed. They will also decide what form of monitoring there should be for these patients and when they should come off the drug. That's now all down to the Prescribing Committee, although the actual decisions on individual cases are still being made by the ECR Committee. The same sorts of procedures apply to new technologies. We are really trying to be more evidence-based and explicit in our decisions than we have been in the past. I actually think we're more explicit than most health authorities.

The more that I become involved in it, the more I think that we have to make value judgments; and there isn't a simple way of trading off different values. We've spent a lot of the last year developing explicit values for this health authority – accessibility, efficacy, effectiveness and so on. But you can't trade off these different values in different contexts and expect to come out with exactly the same answer every time. In practice it just doesn't work. There's always uncertainty and individuality. Randomized controlled trials tell you one thing, but real live doctors are having to make individual clinical decisions as they go along in as scientific a way as they can manage. I don't mean that dismissively, because I think it's quite a good way of doing it. The two don't fit easily together, and if you want to make people change, you have to bear in mind how they really behave.

We've also got to explain it all to the public, and I think we're doing quite well on that. When we were developing our surgical exclusion policy, we were brave enough to say that we weren't buying certain operations, and I continued to say that we weren't buying them even when things got hostile. The media coverage in this instance was really interesting. They generally can't cope with a complex story, but I must say I was pleased at the amount of detail that we got them to go into. But sometimes they couldn't cope with the complexity of it and they said to me, we can't put all of that lot in – we can see it's really complicated and because you've just explained it to us we're going to write a sympathetic piece, but we're not going to put all of that stuff in.

It's important to keep trying, though. The big cases that hit the national press, like little Jaymee Bowen, certainly do arouse a lot of public interest. But what I want to ask is: where are the advocates for all the people who *don't* get treated if a lot of money is spent on high-profile cases? Jaymee was an attractive little girl and I'm very sorry for what happened to her, especially perhaps for the way she was dragged through the papers. But what about all the other people? There's a vast army of them. If the money had been spent on Jaymee, others would not have been treated. Some of them may have been old people needing chiropody or hip replacements or incontinence pads. They don't look as attractive on the front page of our newspapers, but they're important people as well.

We do need to find ways of getting the public involved in these kinds of decisions. It's a democratic society and in the end it is the taxpayers who pay my wages. What I do with their money must be consistent with what they want. But I don't think we can just present the questions to them in an undiluted form. Take the work that was done in North London about the values that people put on paediatric care. Everyone wanted high-tech neo-natal cots and nobody wanted vaccinations. Well, that's silly, and if they had really understood the issues they shouldn't have been saying that. But I don't know how we make them understand. I don't know about that at all. And how far do you slavishly follow what the public tell you they want? I do feel that people should be better informed, but what if they still prefer cuddly little babies to unattractive people with mental illness or learning difficulties? What do we do then? I really don't have an easy answer to that.

The psychiatrist's story

The first point to make is that rationing is not abnormal. It's always been intrinsic to the provision of health care and it is independent of the method by which it's funded. And it's not just the NHS: rationing is equally inevitable in privately funded systems of health care. What is important is the extent of rationing and the way it is carried out. I would say that the public consciousness of rationing has altered in the last few years and it's clearly become a matter of political concern. Although it would be true to say that rationing has only recently emerged as an issue, I think it's been there all the time.

The public are more concerned about it now because of the pace of change, particularly in high-technology secondary care which promises a very great deal for small numbers of patients at a very high cost in some cases. This is clearly quite different from the aim of the NHS in 1948, which was to deliver a high volume of low-cost interventions. So there has been a change in the technology of medical care which has brought the issue of rationing to the public mind much more forcibly, and that in turn has made it a political issue. But the underlying issue of rationing – I wouldn't even go so far as to call it a problem – has always been there. It is absolutely implicit in any system which is providing personal services, not just health care.

From my own perspective as a psychiatrist, rationing affects me most in personnel matters. There never seem to be quite enough colleagues – nurses, social workers, and all the multi-disciplinary members of mental health teams. They all seem to be very busy all of the time, and I think the pressure has been exacerbated by a great many early retirements. That's not unique to the NHS, of course: it has also affected the teaching profession and others as well. There is an expectation nowadays that people will retire earlier and will have more leisure time in the last part of their lives. But this has happened at the very time when the context and the details of health care have become more sophisticated. For example, the level of documentation that is now required is far higher than it was ten years ago. Care plans and supervision registers and various aspects of Mental Health Act administration are all very much more detailed and time-consuming than they once were. And they all involve an opportunity cost in terms of the time we can spend in face-to-face contact with our patients. We have moved in the last 10–15 years from a situation where there were more patient contacts with a relatively low level of documentation and recording, to one where we now have fewer contacts which are exceptionally well documented. One has to ask whether that's necessarily an advance or not.

I can give you quite a graphic example of this. A few days ago one of the consultants in my Trust got in touch with me to say that a mental health review tribunal had required him to give evidence concerning the detention of one of his patients. The tribunal had set a time for the hearing which clashed with an out-patient clinic where he was booked to see five new patients. So he told the tribunal that he was very sorry, but he would be unable to attend at such short notice. The tribunal replied that they would subpoena him and they also hinted that he might be guilty of contempt of court. Well, this is a fairly new development. Until quite recently, tribunals showed a lot of flexibility in fitting in with the clinical pressures on the consultants, but they have now changed their procedure. Why? Because in two or three cases which have recently gone to the European Court, the Court has ruled that a delay in a tribunal hearing might constitute a breach of Article 5 of the European Convention of Human Rights.

So that's a very good example, and my consultant colleague did indeed have to cancel his out-patient clinic and the five new patients will now have to wait several more weeks before they get any medical attention. Of course I can see the other side as well. The human rights of the patient who was detained also had to be safeguarded, and rightly so. It's a value judgment as to where the balance should lie, and I think that value judgments should be debated openly and made explicitly. They shouldn't be introduced by stealth, which is how they actually get introduced into the health service most of the time. So yes, this is rationing, and again it comes down to the opportunity costs that are involved. But it's not something that ever gets a public airing, and I would be very interested to know what public opinion thinks would be the right course of action in a case like this.

You also have to take account of the value judgments of the clinicians who are involved. In this particular case, the comments of my colleague were really rather interesting. He knew the likely risk of missing the tribunal, namely, that he might be subject to adverse criticism and that his detained patient might be denied re-access to a tribunal. On the other hand he *didn't* know the possible risks of not seeing the five new patients. They may all get better by the time they eventually have an appointment to see him, and they may not even turn up; but some may try to harm themselves or even commit suicide. So he was in a difficult position: he could take a sensible view about the risks of one course of action while the risks of the other course of action were almost completely unknown. The difficulty for him is that if one of those five patients harms himself, then the consultant might be found to have been negligent. The general principle is that there are risks involved in taking action and there are risks involved in not taking action; and that's what rationing is all about. But before you can do it properly, you must know exactly what all the risks are.

We're moving now into the territory of clinical judgment, of course. Traditionally, doctors have made their own choices about how they are going to treat their patients, and nobody has asked too many questions about what they are doing or why they are doing it. But we know that clinicians don't necessarily make their choices rationally. When faced with a choice between treatment A and treatment B, a clinician's judgment might be influenced by, for instance, what he used last time or what he feels most comfortable using. He may not want to use treatment B because he's never used it before and he doesn't necessarily know what the side effects are. But it seems obvious to me that the choice between two courses of treatment should be based on the evidence that we have about their effectiveness. This is what evidence-based medicine is all about. To rely on 'clinical judgment' is no more rational than the clinical judgment itself.

I think that these are essentially political matters in the widest sense – not party political, of course – and I think that public policy ought to be determined in the final event by the public. I'm sure that the public can understand the basic idea that one type of treatment may be superior to another in a particular situation, and that the choice between them has implications for the cost to the NHS. There ought to be some way of involving those who are going to receive the treatment as well as those who are going to give it. Take, for example, the advent of new drugs like Donepezil, which has been shown to have a moderately beneficial effect in the short term in the treatment of Alzheimer's disease. The problem is that these drugs are very expensive. And so the question arises of whether it is better to spend our resources on such drugs or in some other way? We've had no opportunity to debate this question because Donepezil is now available and there is a huge public pressure from carers and relatives for their loved ones to be receiving it. I can understand that. On the other hand, some patients may actually be better off receiving more frequent visits at home from a psychiatric nurse or being treated in other ways. The point is that relatives and carers often aren't told about the alternatives and we don't have a debate about them. We just rely on clinical judgment. But I don't think that clinical judgment can help us much here. It's a fig leaf for our own unwillingness as a society to make difficult decisions.

Part of the problem is that doctors are unwilling to relinquish their clinical judgment and therefore their part in the rationing process. And up to a point that is right. The contributions of clinicians will always be needed in rational decision-making about treatments. But what I am saying, I think, is that it is unhelpful and unwise to leave it entirely to clinicians because they don't make these decisions on a strictly rational basis. It may be that the wider involvement of the public wouldn't increase the rationality either; but as I have already said, at least it would bring in those who are going to receive the treatments instead of just those who are going to give them. But generally, there are few signs that clinicians are prepared to stop taking these decisions unilaterally on behalf of their patients. That's their job, and they're always happy to find reasons why their particular patients should be treated differently from anyone else's. This, incidentally, is one of the difficulties in the use of treatment protocols. It's perfectly possible to have sensible guidelines and protocols that we can all agree: the devil lies in the let-out clauses. Everybody is in favour of general parsimony and particular expenditure – their own, that is! That's human nature. We've recently taken over the management of extra-contractual referrals from the health authority, and whenever I get a request to authorize an ECR there is always some particular reason put forward by the referring doctor as to why this should be an exception to the rule. No doubt I'd do it myself. So I'm a little bit suspicious about clinicians who say, OK I'll abide by the rules – until they're applied to me.

Cost is important as well, but I think it is variable between specialties. In my particular specialty – unlike the high-technology specialties – it hasn't been addressed very much. Most of the costs in psychology and psychiatry are in human resources. The cost of drugs and physical treatments is proportionately less, though it is becoming more important as the unit costs of certain drugs begin to rise. But no, costs haven't been to the forefront of clinical thought in my specialty, even when they should have been. An example of this is the wholesale introduction of SSRI anti-depressants in place of the older and much cheaper tri-cyclics. That has now happened. It's an irreversible change that clinicians drifted into without a huge amount of rational thought; and if any rational thought had been given to the cost implications, then I don't think it would have happened. You can see it happening also to a certain extent with newer, more expensive anti-psychotic drugs, which again all clinicians are very keen to use because of the benefits they perceive from them; but they don't perceive the disbenefits which result from the fact that these drugs cost three or four times as much. I'm aware that cost considerations have been taken on board in other specialties, particularly in things like renal medicine where they're using drugs like Erythropoietin which are astonishingly expensive and where its cost could cripple all other workings of the department if it was used indiscriminately. So it's quite a patchy picture.

At the same time, of course, we have to recognize that clinical practice has changed a great deal. Twenty or thirty years ago the number of drugs available for the treatment of mental illness was probably only a quarter of those available today, and they were considerably less effective. This meant that a lot of psychiatrists and other professionals working in mental health were concentrating on psychological interventions simply because there was nothing better. Now, in many cases – though not all, of course – effective biological treatments are available which mean that you don't have to spend an hour, or classically fifty minutes, face-to-face with a patient in one session. Fifteen or twenty minutes, combined with an effective drug treatment, can now achieve just as much as an hour or more might have done twenty years ago. So we would have to take that into account as well.

The question of training doctors and other clinicians about their role in rationing is interesting. My strong impression is that the whole idea of rationing is thought to be slightly indecent to the professional mind. I don't myself subscribe to that view because I began by saying that I think it's absolutely intrinsic to all health care. We do talk about it, of course, but we don't like to do it in front of the patients. It might upset them. That's the general feeling. And the managers might be upset as well! This happened to me quite recently in a conversation with our health authority on our 'care planning' approach and its integration with the social services equivalent of 'case management'. It so happens that the criteria for case management in the local social services department are much clearer and require a higher degree of need than the criteria for our care planning approach. The health authority is extraordinarily reluctant – and I would assume that the same would apply to the Department of Health and to the government – to introduce tighter criteria for care planning. But that's not true in the context of personal social services, and it seems to me illogical that it shouldn't apply in health as well. When I raised this issue, it was quite clear that nobody wanted to talk about it. It was thought to be embarrassing to point out that perhaps the emperor had no clothes. So no, it's not an issue that we as a profession are terribly interested in, and it's not one in which we receive very much training.

We'll never solve the issue of rationing. I'm quite clear about that.

We've been living with it since 1948 and I'm sure we will have to go on living with it for the next 50 years. There is a creative tension arising, it seems to me, from the fact that the supply of health care will never equal the demand for it. That much is quite clear, and there will therefore always be a debate on how to use the resources of the NHS most effectively. And this is where the most difficult ethical questions come in. For myself, I don't think that it is ethical to expend resources on health care that is not going to be effective. That's the way I would put it rather than to go along with what Ivan Illich described as 'equal access to torts' — the idea that everybody should have fair shares of ineffective treatment. I don't go along with that at all, although I guess it is a legitimate ethical perspective.

These are matters of judgment that are essentially political in nature, and I am uncomfortable with the idea that judgments of this sort should be delegated to a particular professional group, as though they could be solved by some special technique of rationality which only that profession can exercise. I prefer to see them as judgments that should involve everyone who has a stake in health care. Ethics is not just about what you do: it's also about how you do it. We need to encourage more open discussion in public. When a health authority decides not to fund, say, gender reassignment surgery or breast augmentation, there's no way at present for the public to be involved. The public may be there at the health authority meeting, but the issue will have been signed and sealed long before that. So the debate takes place in a relatively enclosed professional space and in an atmosphere in which everyone is afraid of controversy. We mustn't rock the boat. We mustn't kick up a fuss. I disagree. I think we should rock the boat and we should kick up a fuss. It's much more mature to have a healthy level of dissent around these things.

The general practitioner's story

I decided to go into fund-holding with some reluctance because I thought it was ethically unsound. When you become a fund-holding practice you believe that it is a better system, and that means that non-fund-holding practices are disadvantaged. Patients who are registered with those practices have absolutely no choice, or only very little choice, because they don't really realize what's going on.

An early and unpleasant example involved physiotherapy. We had a contract at the hospital for physiotherapy which required our patients to be seen within four weeks. If the hospital defaulted, we would not pay. So we told our patients that if they didn't get an appointment in that time, they were to let us know. Well, quite a number of patients told us they were waiting more than four weeks; and so we would phone the hospital and speak to the senior physiotherapist who I suspect didn't believe in fund-holding. It really irked him that he was having to cancel other patients, often patients within the hospital, in favour of ours. He did it with bad grace and I don't blame him one bit. It made me feel awkward about doing it. So we started to employ our own physiotherapist here. It was easier, and morally it was pleasanter to do that.

So that's an example of how, in a way, the system affected us morally. It made us feel guilty and then we made a change as a result. The moral basis is that people's access to services should be determined neither by money nor by an artificial contract but by need. I know that somebody, somewhere, has got to make choices, but I think in this example it is the physiotherapist who should be able to say 'look, we've got this person who has just had a stroke and she needs to have intensive physiotherapy, but there's also this person who has a tennis elbow and all he needs is a bit of ultrasound. He can go way down the list or even pay for it.'

It's the rigidities of the budgeting mechanism that prevent this sort of flexibility, and I feel unhappy about it. I think it creates all sorts of ethical tensions. For instance, we run in-house clinics for surgery, gynaecology and dermatology, and our patients prefer to be seen here because the surgeons come down from the hospital. It's providing a good service for our patients. But I suspect it's at the disadvantage of the non-fund-holding practices. Our patients get seen more quickly in our clinics and then they are put on a waiting list. I presume they have jumped the NHS queue.

I do believe in Aneurin Bevan's principle at the inception of the NHS that need should come before cost. The problem is that when it comes down to it, the general practitioner has a very important role as the advocate for his own patients. Suppose you have a general practitioner who is very conscientious, very hard-working, pushes a lot and feels that the only consideration is the patient sitting there. He sees that patient's need as a real and paramount one. If he refers the patient to the hospital and the appointment comes back for nine months hence, then of course that doctor would feel he's got to write another letter or he's got to phone the secretary and say, this is not good enough. And this is happening more and more. General practitioners nowadays are pushing hard. It's no longer a question of writing one referral letter. You often write two, sometimes three, and a phone call, sometimes two or three phone calls to push hard at the door to get the patient seen when you think is reasonable.

And on the receiving end of this are the consultants who can see what sort of patients they are getting. They inevitably put a loading on some GPs' referrals compared with others. You get a reputation for being either a good judge of what is acute and necessary or one who just worries about anything at all. There is also the ethically worrying aspect to it that if you refer quite a number of patients privately, that consultant will probably see your referrals a little more quickly. That's a little under-hand, but we all know it happens. It's part of our tactics to keep the important consultants happy. I've got friends who are terribly con-scientious about this sort of thing who say they couldn't behave like that. In a way I admire them for it, but I have to say that it always surprises me because it's disadvantaging their own patients. In the end it's a bit like a court of law – you know, it's the advocate who pushes hardest, who is the most persuasive, who wins the day. It's not the truth that matters. I find that a difficult dilemma.

I never used to be an advocate of private care and I don't know whether I still am a non-advocate of it; but it does change your attitude, because you know that if you refer a patient privately it doesn't come out of your budget. So in a way, ironically, you are pleased that they are private patients and you send them up the road, even though you suspect that some surgeons and physicians must be taking time out from their NHS work to see their private patients. But I've no way of knowing that! Anyway, I always ask patients about private insurance when I refer them and it does make me feel slightly uncomfortable. Obviously the longer you've been in general practice, the more you get to know your patients and the more you know who are the arch-communists who would feel angry about being asked. Yes, you feel that it's a slightly uncomfortable question to ask, but you just get hardened to it.

Part of the difficulty is that there's no forum where the GPs can meet with the consultants to discuss these sorts of issues and see if between us we can work out a better way of doing things. There is a Clinical Liaison Committee, but that's really looking at better ways of writing referral letters or conveying information between consultants and GPs. It's not really looking at the ethical issues about referral. Of course you talk to your partners in the practice, but basically you're having to work things out for yourself and pacify your own conscience. We do put on ethical days or half-days where we discuss things like this and we do get people in, specialist people, to talk about medical ethics. So from that point of view I feel that I'm aware of the ideas that are currently floating around. But having said that, I never sit down with other colleagues or con-sultants to talk about particular ethics or intentions.

You always have this sense at the back of your mind, in your day-today work as a GP, that if you give this kind of treatment to this patient, or if you bring in these kinds of services for that patient, then you won't be able to do this, this and this. It's an everyday mindset now. It never used to be, though I do think it was coming in even before fund-holding. Gradually you realized that money wasn't limitless. Now, of course, we're in the great biochemical age of medicine where therapeutics have really taken off. When I first qualified there was a very limited range of drugs we could use. Now there are thousands of them and some of them are extremely expensive, so we consciously worked out some sort of formulary. We looked at the cheaper forms of drugs, and about 50 per cent of our prescribing is now generic.

The big problems crop up with the very expensive drugs. About three years ago I had a patient who I thought had Alzheimer's disease. I sent him to a consultant and the diagnosis came back that it was fairly likely to be Alzheimer's. The consultant knew of a trial of a very new drug, Aricept, and suggested that the patient might like to participate in it. As it happened, there turned out to be some slight doubt whether the patient really had Alzheimer's, so he was excluded from the trial. But the professor who was running the trial wrote back to me saying that he was fairly sure about the diagnosis and that the patient would probably benefit from the drug. He thought it would be reasonable for me to prescribe it when it eventually got its licence. So I did, for about a year, and the patient definitely improved. But then we had a letter from the health authority saying that they would not sanction any more prescriptions for Aricept. By then I had already written about 9–10 months' worth of the drug and I carried on for another two months. After that the patient deteriorated rather rapidly and is now in a home.

Prescribing raises many ethical dilemmas. When we knew that we were going to become fund-holding, we realized that our therapeutics budget would be set by our current spending. So we carried on prescribing in exactly the same way that we always had, and sometimes even a bit more expensively. And once we became fund-holding we had a pretty good idea that whatever profit we had made in our first year would be cut from the following year's budget by a comparable amount. So we decided that we wouldn't change the formulary all at once. If we did, the next year's budget would be cut quite drastically. So we did it in bits. We controlled the change to generic prescribing and now we're up to 50 per cent generic. It's all a bit absurd and artificial. If you told all the GPs in the country that they could keep a quarter of one per cent of whatever money they saved from prescribing, the NHS would be saved billions; and yet we don't do that, and I can't think why the government doesn't do it.

There are effective forms of medical and surgical care that perhaps we ought not to be making available on the NHS at all. In a sense they are at the margins of people's lives. They're not life-threatening and they don't even affect the quality of life in a major way. If people want them, that's fine, but they should pay privately for them, not expect the cost to come from the public purse. Tattoo removal is one. Sterilization operations have gone as well, both male and female. You can't get those under the NHS any more. In vitro fertilization is another example. We've limited that, I suppose arbitrarily, to two menstrual cycles, and after that the couples have to go privately. We looked at the number of people who were demanding IVF and how much we could afford to spend on it, and we said right, two cycles and that's it. In a way, I think this is a benefit of fund-holding. It gives you the leverage to say look, this shouldn't be done under the National Health Service, we don't have a budget for it, and if you disagree with us you must contact your MP. It's a political decision, not a medical one.

I'll give you an example. A young chap in his late 20s was worried that he had bat ears. He had always been embarrassed by them but now he wanted to get something done, and asked me if I would refer him. I said well, we don't have a budget for this type of thing, and although I will refer you, you will have to pay for it yourself. He didn't have private insurance, but as he was in a reasonably well-paid job he had to go privately. Now that was not really an ethical dilemma but it is an example of the way that fund-holding has changed our practice. Cost has come in and it has overridden need. In this case it was ethically acceptable. I mean, I can't get into the mind of the chap and see how he might agonize over his ears even at the age of nearly 30. But I do know that there may well be a lot of patients who have got some disfiguring problem and who genuinely need cosmetic surgery, and we need our limited budget for them.

But there's a problem. If you've run a tight ship and at the end of the year you have made a profit, which we have done year on year, you feel you've done well. You've made a profit of £40,000. But you've done it by not treating patients you could have treated. And then you realize that in fact it's only a paper exercise, so you say, well, if we don't spend the money on something, we're going to lose it; and then you start thinking, what can you spend the money on? It's difficult spending £40,000 just like that on health care, so you tend to spend it in easier ways. For example we bought a hyfrecator and a cryotherapy gun when we started a dermatology clinic – this is something that pulses electric sparks onto warts. We also bought a sterilizer and fridges for inoculations. These all produce medical benefits, but I often wonder whether the money could have been better spent if we had really had the time to plan it and if we had a longer budget allocation – say five years.

We also bought a lot of new computers and all the things that go with them, so now we've got computers till they're coming out of our ears. Can you believe it? Have you any idea how much this practice will have spent on computers by the end of this year? A hundred thousand pounds. Multiplied around the country that's a huge amount of money that could have been spent on health. On the other hand, the computers do make us work more efficiently. In fact I can give you an example of how it can save life. A woman patient had breast cancer and then had a pain in the neck. It could easily have been disc trouble, but because you could see instantly that she had had breast cancer a few years previously, I was able to say I think we ought to get an X-ray straightaway. It does have a beneficial effect. It's something you can really put your finger on. But it is very costly. You often wonder sometimes whether the money could be better spent.

Time is the perennial problem. I can well imagine that the GP's time will become ever more precious because we are all stretched. For instance, I would say that 20 years ago it was fairly common for GPs to be relatively free in the afternoon between 2.00 and 4.00 to mow the lawn, sit in the garden, relax or whatever. Most GPs of my age look back on those heady days. But it's not like that any more. Theoretically, I have a half-day a week off, which happens to be today, but I'm not sure I will see much of it. These days you can only get through all your work by cutting out things like lunch, or having lunch on the hoof, or by cutting out the afternoon leisure time which has long since gone in any case. Some GPs are getting increasingly grumpy about it all. Certainly quite a lot of the older ones are burnt out and have taken early retirement. The point is that we are becoming busier and busier because we are having to provide more and more information for this, that and the other, and we have to collect it and keep it. And consultation times are increasing. I think the average nationally is now around about ten minutes a patient, whereas it used to be six minutes. I know my average is longer than that – it'll be anywhere between three minutes at the very shortest to an hour at the longest. The amount of work that we do in that time has increased because of the speed of the computer. Once you've got it up and running, it does free up your time. Even with a simple thing like writing out a prescription, you can get it clattering away and you can then be carrying on the consultation with the patient. You can certainly make more out of your time. There are undoubtedly benefits. But it is at a cost.

There's no doubt that there is a certain section of the profession that has become increasingly brassed off about the current state of general practice, but on the other hand there are those who do feel the excitement of all the changes and the benefits they have brought. I'm nowhere near burnt out. There are times when I get fed up, but it's only because I've just got too much to do and I just can't do it. I would love to be able to go into research, but I can't do it. I couldn't possibly contemplate doing that sort of thing because of the time involved. I've written a couple of books, but you're having to do that late at night; and as far as audit work is concerned, that's just not possible. I think it's what the state wants us to do, but they will have to find more GPs in order to free up time, because at the moment they're giving us more and more and more work.

The geriatrician's story

For me, rationing exists whenever there is any constraint that stops me from providing a service in the way that I think it should be provided. If I could do something in a better way, but I'm prevented from doing so by a constraint on resources, then I will regard that as rationing. That's how I look at it, and I think that all clinicians would recognize it in their work – hour by hour if not actually minute by minute. It's obviously a fundamental constraint under which we work.

Take the matter of time, for example. It's quite clear as one goes through one's daily work that one can't allocate the time that one would like to give to the clinical care of each individual patient. Time is constrained and limited, and in the ideal situation one would like to spend a lot more time with each patient, both on an in-patient basis and, equally, in the out-patient clinics. When you're faced with these kinds of pressures on your time you have to prioritize your work. Clinical care obviously comes first. On the out-patient side, we try to impose some sort of structure so that the numbers of patients don't just run away. We see a fairly consistent number of patients in each clinic because we have to balance the demands for consultations against what one would ideally like to do in that clinic. So one still sees more patients than one would want to see ideally, but that is the only way you can keep the waiting time for the clinic down to a reasonable level. On the in-patient side, the work is much more variable. A lot depends on the number of patients who are in the hospital, and you simply have to work around that. You give whatever time you have available.

The other problem with time, of course, is that the clinical role has grown steadily, and there are all sorts of additional things that one is now expected to do such as teaching, training, audit, research and so on. I think the teaching and the training are particularly demanding, and consultants these days are having to give up far more of their time to make sure the junior staff are properly trained. It is totally understandable and very reasonable, but it does have a major impact on how you get through the workload. Demands of this sort creep in without your noticing them, and then you have to adjust your job plans and work arrangements to accommodate them. As the pressures build up, though, it's increasingly difficult trying to fit them all in, and in fact the Royal College of Physicians has just produced a document indicating what they think is a reasonable workload. I find it extremely useful in identifying the problem and in trying to arrive at a sensible workload that will ensure the provision of adequate care. It would be helpful if we could all move towards that sort of thing.

So time is certainly very much one factor, not just for doctors but for everyone. You've only got to look at the ward teams to realize that we don't have enough nurses for the work that needs to be done, and they are extremely limited in what they can do for each individual patient. They've got two key roles: they've obviously got to care for the patient but they've also got to contribute to the rehabilitation of the patient; and while they may have just about enough time to provide adequate care, it's very hard for them to find the time to meet the rehabilitation goals that we're trying to achieve. So yes, I am sure they would say that their time is limited.

The same is true for the therapists. For instance, our physiotherapists calculated recently that the average length of time that patients get for physiotherapy is ten minutes a day. Well, in an active rehabilitation unit that can't really be ideal, and we're actually quite well staffed in physiotherapy compared to many other units. So that's an indication of the amount of physiotherapy you get on the NHS when you need rehabilitation, and it's not a great deal. We've just been doing a study here to see whether more physiotherapy would make a difference in terms of rehabilitation progress, and our impression is that if we could give more than ten minutes it would make a difference. Obviously we don't know the precisely ideal amount of physiotherapy that patients would benefit from, but I suspect it's more than ten minutes.

The facilities that are available to us in our work is another key area where there are constraints and rationing. You only have to glance around the wards in which the elderly are cared for to appreciate that they're not being cared for in an ideal environment and that the actual structure of the building is inappropriate for the quality of service that we're trying to provide. That's not in any way a reflection on the actual services provided or on the care that we give but on the buildings themselves – their layout, the access to toilets, the number of beds in a ward. They're all far from ideal, and because the money isn't forthcoming to replace them, it does represent a form of rationing of services. In an ideal situation one wouldn't want to provide the service in the structures that we have here.

I'm trying to think of examples where rationing does not occur, and that's almost harder! But yes, there are certain areas, like for instance drug treatment and equipment, where I feel there is really no rationing at all. In geriatric medicine we use a lot of relatively inexpensive drugs as opposed to a few extremely expensive ones, and I suppose for that reason we don't come up against the issue of the rationing of drug treatment in the way that, say, oncology or renal medicine does. It's true that there is a costly new drug for Alzheimer's disease, but to my mind it is still at the stage of being evaluated. It doesn't yet have an established place in clinical practice and we don't know who are the right patients to prescribe it for or under what conditions. The recommendation that we have received is that patients who might be suitable for the drug should be referred to a professional psycho-geriatrician who would properly assess them, and that is what I do. I certainly wouldn't reckon to prescribe it myself in a routine way. So I can't say that my use of it is rationed. Otherwise I would say that every patient gets what is judged to be appropriate for them, and I think that would probably go for equipment as well. You have to remember that we don't use equipment very intensively, certainly not costly equipment, and so we do have most of what we want.

You ask whether these various constraints are affecting core standards of care or only the peripheral things like comfort and satisfaction. It reminds me of a visit that we had a few years ago from the Chief Executive of the Health Authority when we were trying to reorganize the service. We were explaining the sort of service that we felt we should be providing, and he said, you can't expect to have a Rolls Royce service, you must accept the Mini Minor service. Well, that filled us all with great gloom and despondency, but I guess one can see the point. Are we striving merely to provide the bare minimum that's acceptable? Are we trying to provide a good service? Or are we trying to provide a Rolls Royce service? I think one could accept that it's probably over-ambitious to go for the Rolls Royce service, but I do think we should be aiming at more than a Mini Minor service. At the moment, I personally feel that we could be providing better care. Our care is adequate, it's reasonable even, but it's sometimes pretty close to the bare minimum. I feel we are constantly being driven by the need for efficiency in whatever we do. There's a constant increase in the number of patients coming through and we're always having to watch the bed situation. So yes, there has been this drive for efficiency which has pushed us very close to what I think of as an acceptable standard, and I would certainly like to see more time available to provide a more considered management regime for a larger number of patients.

On the acute side, certainly, the pressure of patients coming through is obviously a national problem. From one point of view it's reassuring that it's not just our local problem. We would be worried if we felt something strange was happening in our particular hospital. But it does put us under enormous pressure to be getting patients out of hospital really as soon as their feet touch the accident and emergency department or the medical assessment unit. Often over the last two or three years I've regarded myself almost as a discharge machine, which is really not the way it should be; but the moment patients arrive in the hospital you find yourself thinking, how can we get them back into the community as quickly as possible? And of course one can justify it in various ways. There are all sorts of problems with being in hospital, and it's much better if people are in the community. But nevertheless, I can't help feeling sometimes that this is only a rationalization, and that the real reason is to make the services as efficient as possible.

I do sometimes feel that we are actually pushing for too much efficiency at the expense of high-quality care. This is obviously a very delicate issue, but I suspect that it really does affect clinical care. Of course, it depends what outcomes you look at. You could look, for instance, at the number of medications that patients are on, particularly in the older age groups, and whether this is ideal. Unless you have enough time to assess a patient's situation thoroughly and know their clinical background and so on, it's all too easy for them to end up on the wrong mixture of drugs. Often they will end up on more drugs than are really necessary for them. They may get to the situation where one drug is prescribed to counter the side-effects of another and you are then into poly-pharmacy. That's one kind of outcome. A different kind of outcome – a functional one – would be to look at patients' capacity to be as independent as possible. Unless elderly people are given the time to be thoroughly evaluated, some of their conditions can be missed or over-looked, and then you end up with somebody more dependent than they would otherwise be. Well, those are some examples of where clinical care could be improved.

What is happening in situations like this is that long-term problems are being stacked up for the sake of short-term budgetary savings. I often think that our efficiency might be greater overall if we were able to spend more time making very thorough and effective evaluations in the first place because I believe we would actually save more money in the long term. One reason why we don't go down this road is that the savings would be hard to prove, and I'm not sure whether it has ever been done. But I think the main reason is that we have been driven by the overriding need for the acute hospitals to reduce their costs. The managers are constantly trying to stop elderly patients from getting into their acute hospitals at all, and then try to get them out again as quickly as possible. Yet this is precisely the environment in which the elderly need to be thoroughly assessed because it's in the acute hospital that the more complicated investigations are done and it's there that you've got all the specialist advice you might want. Look at the community hospitals – they usually have a lot of elderly patients who have been there for quite long periods of time, but in many cases the length of stay in the community hospital could have been significantly reduced if they had been investigated more aggressively in the acute hospital at the outset. And the fact that they are not comes back to the enormous costs of acute hospital care. That's the theory, at least. It would be extremely interesting to test it.

You ask where ethical notions fit into all of this – whether one is always consciously trying to allocate time and other facilities in relation to patients' needs. Well, my answer is no. The idea that one patient is more in need than another and should therefore get more of the time of the doctor or the nurse or the therapist does not have any great resonance for me. It doesn't actually work like that. It may be because of the nature of this particular work. The elderly tend to present with fairly non-specific complaints and many of them have multiple pathologies, so it would be hard to judge whether some should have more time than others. To me it's more a question of continual cohorts of patients coming through and you have just got to try to do the best you can for each of them in turn. I don't feel in any way that I am trying to deny something to one patient in order to give more to another. It's more a question of having time to cope with all of them coming through. There's a constant weight of people coming through, and you know that you have got to move them on and out so that you can make space for the next ones who will be coming through the front door.

What we mustn't do, though, is to create a formal rationing system that could work against the interests of the elderly. As a geriatrician, I have always been trying to defend the rights of this disadvantaged group and I have been battling against any formal rationing of services for the elderly for a long time. I see it as our role to push those barriers back rather than to create or reinvent any new ones. We're always trying to get more resources – not necessarily vast resources for highly expensive treatments, but reasonable resources for the things that work. In an environment where you're constantly being told that you must become more efficient and save more money, we know that our resources will be cut unless we're always testing the barriers and pushing them back as far as we can. If we don't do that, then the geriatric service will suffer. So that's been the practical line that we have adopted – well, that I've adopted – and I haven't allowed myself to worry too much about the overall cost.

In fact, I think the country is actually getting quite a reasonable health service at a very cheap rate, and there's a lot of scope for putting a bit more money into the pot and seeing what sort of improvements you can get from it. That would be true of the service as a whole, but it would be particularly true from the point of view of the elderly because their requirements are not especially expensive. All they need is access to what are now pretty standard investigations – CT scanning, MRI, and things like that which really are generally accessible nowadays and in fact are regarded as routine. There certainly shouldn't be any kind of rationing or ring-fencing around these sorts of services. To me, if there is to be any form of control or limitation on people's access to care it should be through some form of insurance against major disasters such as renal failure. I know it's very unlikely to happen and I have no idea what level of insurance payments would be involved; but it does seem to me in principle that expensive treatments for fairly uncommon conditions may be suitable for some form of insurance.

Ageism is always a problem in the context of rationing. There is a lot of discrimination against the elderly and in fact the elderly are very much against themselves, even though they don't realize it. They are very undemanding and they don't usually realize what can be done for them nowadays. The acceptance of illness and disability among the elderly is really quite remarkable. They think that just because they're getting old, they're bound to be crippled with arthritis or with limited mobility. They see Parkinson's disease as just another feature of old age, whereas of course it's eminently treatable now. So one has to get the message across to them as much as anybody else that there are all sorts of things which can be done and should be done to improve their quality of life and their functional independence. So yes, I still think there's an awful lot more that we could do to ensure that the elderly have a reasonable access to effective care, and I'll keep working to try and achieve that.

But things are probably changing in any case. There's a much more informed generation coming through now where people have higher expectations of health care and they will carry that through into old age. I sometimes wonder whether a greater tolerance of disease and disability is actually built into the ageing process and whether it is this which makes people more accepting of their conditions. It's inevitable that old age will carry an increased risk of conditions that lead to disability, and I do sometimes think that psychological changes may occur that allow us to cope with ill health better than we might have done at a younger age. It always seems to me remarkable how stoically older people put up with real disabilities which younger people wouldn't tolerate, and how they manage to maintain such a reasonable quality and spirit of life. So there may be a psychological adjustment; but nevertheless I suspect we will see that future generations coming through will actually be much more demanding and will expect a better quality of care.

The community psychiatric nurse's story

Yes, I do think that rationing has an impact on the service we can provide. It certainly has an indirect impact on my own work, but that's because much of my work is with social service networks that have been rationed or hit by cuts. When this occurs, then of course it has an effect on the way that we work. Suppose there is an emergency in a family, with social or psychological difficulties that require a social worker's skills – what do you do if there isn't one available? Or again, there may be difficulties in securing a place of safety for children who aren't necessarily covered by the Children Act and who don't really come under the Mental Health Act either. They can fall into a grey area where nobody is really responsible. So yes, I think that rationing has allowed holes to be created in the network of services that should be catching people who need help, and consequently their problems become bigger.

Of course, meetings do take place between the health service and social services. I do know there have been meetings between our directorship and the social services directorship to look at how we can handle the shortfall; but I guess that at the coal-face there is still little co-ordination. There is still a feeling that children, who really are valuable assets, are not getting quite as good a service as they deserve. There are many examples, but I don't particularly want to quote them because of confidentiality. But yes, there are lots of families who need to be supported almost on a daily basis, and we cannot always supply the services they need. There are shortfalls and there are not enough resources; and that has a knock-on effect on the children when they are at school, and their education suffers. I think in a way that as a society we make very negative trade-offs. Perhaps you could call it neglect, because if we don't recognize that there are shortfalls, then we are in danger of creating more and more problems in future generations. I would just like us to recognize when a child is not really getting a very great deal. That's not to say that everyone is not getting a good service, because they are – as far as we can provide it.

I don't think the problem is unique to this area. Everyone is experiencing what is basically a lack of money. Actually, some people would argue that money isn't really the answer and I would agree that, with some of the problems we have to deal with, it isn't the answer. But I also think that if we did have a larger amount of money to focus on particular problems, then we might have more success. In a sense, society should be a good supporting parent for these very deprived families who have experienced trauma or loss in many different aspects of their lives but who have never experienced real concern or been given real support. We do help to provide that kind of support, but we should be doing it better.

I find it difficult to say just how big a problem it is in this particular area. I sometimes think – though it may be a fantasy of mine – that if we had more money, there would be fewer problems; but they would probably just be different types of problems. Even if we had a 25 per cent increase in our budget, it would seem like a drop in the ocean. The irony is that if we had more money, we might find that we were admitting more children to the psychiatric service, and I'm not sure we should be doing that. More money might simply make it appear to be a bigger problem than it really is. If we did more for the children just because we had more money, it could actually increase other difficulties that they have and leave them feeling even less worthy. But in some cases it could make a real difference. For instance, there are times when all that the children need, and their families too, is a bit of breathing space. When there's been a psychological outburst because of the family dynamics or a family trauma, then even if there's a family there, it would be vitally important and it would save this service a great deal by having respite beds just for a night or two. Just to give them time. We do have contracts for a private in-patient service, but it can take three weeks to get access to it even in an emergency, and by that time the problem is either reduced or has taken many different shades.

This sort of thing does affect what you can do as a professional person. Of course it does. When I'm on call I could be very stretched. For example I was out last night until midnight assessing a girl who was possibly suicidal, and I knew that if I started the ball rolling, well . . . In fact she wasn't suicidal. She was incredibly unhappy, but she certainly wasn't suicidal. But later I thought, well, if she had been suicidal, what would I have done, because it would take all night to find a bed. If a child needs that sort of sanctuary, that sort of asylum in the true sense of support, there isn't anywhere readily at hand. Children are vulnerable and they could lose their lives. And that's very hard on you as a person because you know it's the result of a shortfall. I know there are children who are at risk because we don't have adequate ancillary resources or things like respite beds. So yes, it does have an impact on my approach and that is quite frustrating.

I believe that we are starting to feel the thin end of the wedge. Less perhaps than other services, but I think we are beginning to feel it because the wider systems of society have been squeezed and that has a knock-on effect on families – through unemployment, loss, whatever. It affects people's physical health and mental health, and indirectly that raises the profile – or at least the expectations – of the problems we are supposed to deal with. Increasingly, we are dealing more with social problems than psychological and emotional problems. There are more children, I think, experiencing real pressures in their lives nowadays, and I think there are more children feeling suicidal than there were, say, five or six years ago. In my experience there's been a steady increase in the rate of overdoses and threats of suicide. Even though some of them may be para-suicidal, they are expressing a depression that's perhaps been building up for a long time, and they should be taken seriously. And they are taken seriously – every time. But then there are problems in the sense of my own resources to deal with it. It's then that it helps to have a well-established support system. It may not change the external system that much, but at least it acts as a form of barometer to measure my own resources and to build my own priorities. You realize that perhaps you don't have to take that case on this week or that something else is more important. So I do think that in a wider social context, rationing does have an impact on what we do and when and how we do it.

We do have guidelines about what we should be doing within our budgets, but sometimes you have to meet them almost dancing on your feet. When you're working at the coal-face, when you're doing an assessment shall we say, then yes, you are working within guidelines; but you still have to deal with the problems in your own way, and no two problems are quite the same. I'm grateful for a lot of support from my manager, but the managers don't always understand our work. Because of the recent complex changes in this Trust, the managers are having to focus on their part of the system, their own bit of the world, and they don't really realize the difficulties we experience when we are face-to-face with families that are breaking up emotionally. Yes, there is a lack of understanding. They have to deal with the management and the structure of the system and they have difficulty sometimes in relating this to the real lives of families.

For example, I might find myself facing a family which needs social services, really needs them, but social services say they haven't got any money to provide a carer or whatever needs to be done, and they will review it in three months' time. So what can you do? You can either say well, actually it's nothing to do with us, it's really social services; or else you can say – to satisfy your conscience, because of course you're talking about people – that you'll be supporting the family over the next three or four weeks on a daily basis with the idea of hopefully developing a therapeutic strategy to help them to understand what's going on, and then you'll withdraw and monitor the situation. But if we do this, it may mean committing three or four senior people over a period of three or four weeks for one family; and management will say that that's not good costing. But of course it is. To my mind it's extremely good costing. If we can save a child from feeling desperately suicidal, then we have stopped that family from becoming desperate and breaking up and all the other factors that would then come into the equation. It's the difference between a short-term budget and a long-term investment. In the short term we must do things as effectively and efficiently as we can. There's no doubt about that because otherwise we couldn't produce adequate care. But there needs to be more thought about the longer term as well. It's about investment as well as consumption. We have to think about the future as well as the present.

Of course, a lot of what I do is simply fire-fighting. You go where the alarm bells are ringing loudest. I know I do. My professional code of ethical conduct would not allow me to walk away from a situation where a person is in need. But my own personal ethos also leads me to believe that we have to take on all the difficulties as we find them. Whether it is really a social services problem or a health problem may be a moot point, but the thing is that we have to understand – or try to understand – what the problem really is. And then we just have to deal with it. I think my own personal ethos is that everyone is valuable. I just believe, I suppose from my own religious beliefs, that everyone is a valuable human being and everyone is worth working with and everyone is equal and should be equally valued.

Of course, there are times when it is just not possible to treat everyone equally, and then you have to fall back on seeing what is the priority. For example, if a child is in danger, then clearly we have to measure the level at which the child is in danger. If the child is in danger from the parents, then social services must be involved because there is a statutory need for child protection. I think I clearly base my priorities on people's needs. Sometimes, if I haven't enough resources of my own to deal properly with a child in need, I would look at wider possibilities. I may even consider bringing in the police if there is violence or if there are psychological problems that are coming to the point of aggression or destruction. There is no way that I can contain that. I don't expect to be able to, because I have to consider my own safety as well. And then there are children and young people in need where the system is letting them down and it should be better; but you might feel well, perhaps it isn't a really pressing need. So you don't do anything for the time being.

I think there needs to be more public awareness of the whole problem of rationing. Clearly we do need the services that we have now because on the whole they work very well, even though there aren't enough resources. But the government needs to be aware of the difficulties we are working under, and so does society. It needs a double-bladed sword, doesn't it? The public needs to know what is going on so that it can become an issue and be taken on board politically. And the politicians also need to realize that there aren't enough resources for the job we're supposed to do. But what is very, very important in all of this is that the professionals shouldn't be left isolated and high-and-dry, coping with everything on their own and taking the blame when it goes wrong. Everyone has clay feet and no-one can say that they always get it right. I don't think at the end of the day that we do get it right all the time. But I also feel that we sometimes ask too much of the professionals. I know that I feel cautious about my work. Caution is now creeping in to the point where yes, I am becoming more resentful, or probably will become more resentful, because I think that more and more is being asked of us and there doesn't seem to be an end to it. So it is obviously up to ourselves, through our professional bodies, to say hold on, enough is enough. But how can you say that when you see families in distress? That is the difficulty one finds oneself in.

7

Principles, practices and ethics

Principles

That a significant gap exists in developed countries between the level of potential demand for health care and the capacity of the economic system to finance it is now taken almost for granted in the contemporary writings of those who have studied the issues. That the gap can be consciously minimized by squeezing out inefficiencies and by controlling the use of unproven and ineffective procedures is uncontroversial. That a significant gap will remain even after such measures have been taken appears to be inevitable. This much, at least, is largely common ground.

Disputation breaks in as we start to shift from the 'is' to the 'ought' – from 'how the world is' to 'what we should be doing about it'. It is here that principles begin to loom; and principles are based in values; and values are pluralist and contested. On certain questions of principle there does appear to be a measure of agreement. We should, in principle, be making adequate investments in disease prevention and health promotion, partly though not principally in order to moderate the demands that are made upon the curative services. We should, in principle, be seeking to produce and deliver specified packages of care at the least cost – provided the pursuit of efficiency does not impose unacceptable stresses on the staff involved. We should, in principle, ensure that treatments and procedures which are offered to the public have been tested for their effectiveness as well as their safety, and those that are found wanting subjected to some form of control over their use.

Beyond this largely uncontentious domain, however, lie large tracts of deeply contested territory. Should the gap between demand and supply in health care be managed or merely coped with? On the one side are the optimistic rationalists who believe that it is not only desirable but also possible to manage the gap in ways that will bring the distribution of care broadly into line with predetermined patterns of equity and justice. On the other side are the cautious realists who, while not deriding rationalism as a principle, see little scope in the complex plurality of health care for much more than a kind of wise and humane muddling through, in which we should expect no more from those who struggle daily to produce the miraculous quart of care from the pint pot of resources than that they behave with care, discernment and sensitivity.

Should the methods of handling the gap, whatever they may be, be revealed to those whose lives and fortunes may be affected by them? On the one side are the honest democrats, committed to principles of openness and transparency in government, who believe in the right of people to know the *modus operandi* of systems which may affect their own and their family's well-being. Whether the gap is actively managed or merely coped with is of secondary importance. What matters is that people should be given a full and accurate account of the decisions which affect not only their immediate health but possibly their life-chances also. On the other side are the caring paternalists, committed more to what they believe to be the welfare of patients than the transparency of systems, who fear the gratuitous hurt that people may suffer through knowing that their conditions, though treatable in principle, have been passed over largely for economic reasons.

Should the values that are reflected in the way the gap is handled be those of the general public (suitably informed and educated about the issues) or should they be those of the politicians, managers, clinicians and other experts, who not only have a clearer understanding of the issues than the 'average' citizen but who may also carry a measure of responsibility for putting the principles into operation? On the one side are the grass-roots populists, insisting that those who pay the piper must have a clear voice in calling the tune and that, however it is done, the handling of the gap must reflect publicly expressed views and opinions. On the other are the principled elitists, fearful that public opinion may, on crucial issues, deliver the wrong verdict. If public opinion, properly sampled, favours a way of proceeding that breaches established principles of fairness, or if it rejects, say, the care and development of children with learning difficulties in favour of expensive technological care for extremely low birth-weight babies, then it must be set aside.

Should the health service give preference to those who are in the greatest need of care or to those who will benefit most from receiving it? On the one side are the champions of justice, concerned lest the needs of particular patients are swept aside in the headlong quest for ever higher levels of aggregate health among groups of patients. Lives are personal as well as statistical, and priorities should reflect the just claims that individual patients have for clinical care, even if the cost of expensive treatment for one patient is a slippage against a target index of aggregate health for many. On the other side are the modern utilitarians, firm in their belief that, whenever resources are limited, they should be used in ways that produce the greatest amount of welfare for the greatest number of people. It is, they claim, economically inefficient if not actually morally wrong to spend a quantum of resource on the care of one person with a poor prognosis if it is done at the cost of estimable improvements in the health of many.

Should the selection of patients for treatment, in situations where all cannot be treated to the same extent, reflect only the relative intensity of their needs for care, or can other personal features and characteristics also properly be taken into account? On the one side are the ethical individualists, who dismiss the relevance of such personal qualities as age, gender, class, merit, social responsibility, economic value, or anything else. To take account of such extraneous features would be to distort the foundational purpose of the NHS, namely to select patients for treatment on the basis of their clinical need and nothing else. On the other side are the pragmatists, who argue that criteria additional to clinical need may be morally admissible in some (though not in all) circumstances. While there may be no serious case for selecting people on the basis of, say, their gender or ethnicity, it may be fair in certain contexts to take account of their age, the extent of their family and other responsibilities, and possibly their economic and social value to their communities.

Since these disputations involve values about the nature of a just society, they are incapable of resolution. I may feel that it is fair, all else being equal, to favour younger people over older people for treatment; my neighbour may not. We each have our reasons and we can each relate our views to a wider set of principles that we hold about the nature of the good society. We certainly can and should debate our respective positions with the greatest possible clarity and honesty; and as a result, one of us may shift his values and change his position. But this is just about all we can do. Beyond that, we must agree to disagree. Meanwhile, those who manage the NHS and who provide the care it offers must battle round the clock to do the best they can with the resources they are given, conscious of the noise of ethical debate reverberating around them but lacking the time to leave the battle-front and make their contribution to the argument. How do their views and experiences illuminate the intrinsically unresolvable tensions of rationing?

The stories recounted in Chapter 6 are neither comprehensive in the issues they encompass nor typical in the views they project. They are, strictly speaking, representative only of themselves. Yet they do provide an unusually detailed and textured series of insights into the rationing that takes place in the NHS, allowing us to see *a* picture – if not a universal picture – of the real world of care at the coal-face rather than the assumed world of those who merely talk about it from the safety of the pit-head. What can we learn from the stories?

Practices

The ubiquitous gap between supply and demand

First and most obviously, the stories attest to the ubiquity of the gap between supply and demand and hence the need for rationing in one form or another. The language may differ but the sentiment is the same: all the informants felt pressured by the lack of resources of one kind or another, and all were having to make a continuous stream of decisions about priorities in their work. The health visitor described her workload as excessive and her job as almost impossible, forcing her continually to decide which of the many tasks demanding her attention were the most important. The district nurse observed that rationing ran like a con-tinuous thread through her work. The GP remarked that the notion of opportunity cost – what had to be given up if something else was done – was now part of the everyday mindset of himself and his partners. The psychiatrist had no doubt that the excess of demand over supply was intrinsic and unavoidable, and both he and his colleagues seemed always to be very busy. The nurse manager described her clinical nursing colleagues as working right up to the line and sometimes beyond it in terms of managing demands against resources. It was, she confessed, a major headache. Pressure of this kind seems to be normal rather than exceptional, permanent rather than occasional. It is an ever-present feature of the health service rather than a transient phenomenon induced by time-limited events which will eventually pass.

Where the shoe was pinching

The shoe pinched the interviewees in different places. For most, time was the commodity under the greatest pressure. When they spoke of the need to prioritize, it was their professional time to which they were usually referring. The surgeon said, quite simply, that he had too much to get through in a day. He was trying to do too much in the 24 hours and some of his patients were not getting as much of his time as either they or (sometimes) he would like. The geriatrician spoke of time as constrained and limited – not only his own time, but that of other members of the team on whom he relied for the effective care of his patients. He would have liked to spend more time with each patient and he would have liked his rehabilitation patients to have more than ten minutes of physiotherapy a week. The pressures of time upon the community nurses were intensified by the lack of cover when they were on holiday or sick leave. We don't get any extra nurses, said the district nurse, and we just have to stretch ourselves further. For her, time could easily eat into her personal life as she tried to keep abreast of her workload. By contrast, perhaps because of the way in which the flow of patients to him was controlled, time was not a major problem for the neurologist. He seemed able to give sufficient time to his patients. In his case, the shoe pinched in other places.

Drugs, investigations and treatments were, for some interviewees, an important focus of rationing. Expensive drugs were not available for prescription as readily as some of the doctors would have wished. The GP had had to cease the prescription of Aricept for an elderly man with dementia, who then began to deteriorate. The neurologist was unable routinely to prescribe Riluzole, which he described as the only proven drug for the treatment of motor neurone disease. The public health physician found that the prescribing of Beta Interferon had to be negotiated carefully with health authorities and with organizations representing the interests of MS patients. Tests and investigations could also be subject to restrictions. The unpredictable (rather than the chronic) non-availability of certain tests and investigations presented the surgeon with difficult clinical choices. He could find a test was rationed one day but not the next. Sometimes it was predictable and sometimes it wasn't; and whether or not he ordered a test might depend upon his perception of its current availability.

The issues surrounding the availability of treatments rather than drugs or investigations were different. The commissioning manager argued that very few treatments were simply not available on the NHS: in most cases patients get the treatments they need, though they may have to wait for them. The doctors seemed broadly to support this view. Even where treatments had clearly been excluded from the menu of those for which a health authority was prepared to pay, let-out clauses, policed in some way or another by the health authority, had usually allowed exceptional cases to pass through the net. But that was not the whole picture: echoes of more deliberately targeted exclusions were to be heard in the stories. The commissioning manager described the debate currently in train in his locality – and farther afield – about the circumstances in which people might in future be denied access to bypass grafts and angioplasty because of their age; and the surgeon spoke of vascular surgeons sometimes taking the view that the chances of a successful outcome were so low that an operation was not thought to be an appropriate use of resources. In other, more numerous cases, a service which was available in principle was not in practice offered to patients who failed to meet the predetermined criteria. Particularly in community nursing, rationing by qualification appeared to be widely practised by the service managers. Thus, incontinence pads were supplied by the health authority in whose area the district nurse worked – but only to those with debilitating illnesses or continence problems resulting from surgery. Bath aids were provided – but only for those who had had surgery or were terminally ill.

Buildings, equipment and beds were another area where the shoe pinched for some interviewees. The geriatrician was hampered in what he was trying to do by the archaic structures of the hospital in which he was working, and the service given by the community psychiatric nurse would have been much better if a smallish number of respite beds had been available to him when they were needed. Beds were not always available for patients coming into the acute hospitals either, particularly those arriving for day surgery. At times, according to the nurse manager, beds not officially designated for in-patient use had to be pressed into service for this purpose. For those working outside the hospital, the pressures centred more around equipment and services than facilities – often quite mundane equipment like bath aids and hoists in the home, or cheap and unglamorous services like laundering. For the community nurses, in particular, life seemed often to be a tussle between themselves and social services over the acceptance of responsibility for providing a joint service. Rationing that is internal to the NHS is exacerbated by the (sometimes even tighter) rationing of social services departments.

Narrowing the gap

Although the interviewees seemed clearly resigned to the inevitability of rationing as an everyday feature of their professional lives, almost all described elements of the waste and inefficiency they saw around them which, if tackled systematically, might help at least to narrow the gap if not entirely to close it. Some of the perceived waste was bureaucratic in origin: the growth in managerial and financial posts, the time devoted to the collection of statistics, and the time required to be spent in fulfilling the demands of patients' charters. Much of the waste originated in clinical rather than administrative actions, reflecting the lack of incentive systems for doctors to use their resources well. The GP spoke of the deliberately high levels of prescribing that his practice had maintained in the run-up to fund-holding and the less than optimal disposition of end-of-year surpluses. The psychiatrist commented on the rapid and uncritical take-up of new drugs in his specialty and the surgeon confessed to the creeping, unintended growth in the use by consultants of expensive new facilities such as scanning and imaging. The surgeon talked also of the inappropriate use of acute hospital beds resulting from a lack of alternative facilities elsewhere, delays in awaiting the results of tests, difficulties in discharging patients to their homes, and the unpenalized practice of surgeons in blocking beds that they wished to be available to them at future times. Without incentives, as the public health physician found, changes in clinical behaviour can be hard to achieve.

A different kind of waste was reflected in the concern of the community nurses over what they saw as the low investment in preventive care, resulting in higher future costs as problems grew unchecked. The under-investment in families with disabled children was a recurrent theme in the health visitor's story, and the same concern was reflected also in the district nurse's derision of a policy that denied incontinence pads to some elderly patients only to incur higher costs later on for the treatment of sores and skin infections. A wider issue, of which these were merely illustrations, was the perceived inflexibility of operational budgets in the NHS. Managers who controlled the local budgets were often portrayed as out of touch with the detailed conditions at the coal-face and unable or unwilling to respond quickly and flexibly to the need for more spending now in order to save money later. The devolution of at least part of the operational budget to the front-line staff would, in the view of the community nurses, result not only in a better standard of care but also, in the longer term, in budgetary savings as well. In the absence of devolved budgets, the community nurses saw themselves as buffers between their patients and their managers, trying to do the best they could for the former without upsetting the latter. It may only have been her seniority that allowed the district nurse, in some situations, to do what was right for her patients and worry later about accounting for the costs to her manager.

The effects of rationing

The effects of the daily struggle to match needs with resources cannot easily be inferred from the stories. Several interviewees spoke of the effects on themselves and their colleagues. Managing the rationing process at the coal-face is stressful. The district nurse spoke more in resignation than in anger about patients taking out their frustrations on the very staff who were doing their best to assuage them. Less resigned was the nurse manager, who regretted the squabbles that went on between ward managers when beds were in very short supply: there were, she thought, better ways of handling hospital management systems that might reduce the need for turf wars of this kind. Similar battles were waged between health and social services staff over the responsibility for patients with both medical and social needs. The failure to alleviate the stresses experienced by the front-line staff in coping with the struggles of the day-to-day rationing of service resulted, according to the nurse manager, in low morale, high sickness levels, long hours of work, and emotional frustration.

Unacceptable variations in the treatment of different patients were also identified as an undesirable consequence of the way that rationing works. Patients who know how to manipulate the system to their advantage, or who are prepared to throw their weight around, can secure preferential treatment. That, said the surgeon, is how the system works: inevitably, it is to some extent responsive to those who exert the greatest pressure on it. Yet it worried him that the consequence might be, as he put it, that the little old lady in social class four will simply say: oh well, that's how things are, I've got to wait. A similar concern about equity was expressed by the public health physician: cases that are given a high profile in the media may lead to the use of costly treatments on unpromising patients while the needs of old people for hip replacements or chiropody go unmet. A bubbly young child with terminal cancer is much more promising copy for the press than an old lady with a weak bladder. Staff who know how to massage the system may also be able to secure better care for their patients than those who don't – a provider-induced inequity. The district nurse who was confident in her ability to appease her managers over her use of expensive bandages for patients with leg ulcers, and who was prepared to arrange whatever Marie Curie nursing her cancer patients might need and worry later about the costs, was getting a better deal for them than other patients in neighbouring localities.

A different kind of equity issue was raised by the informal collusion of doctors over the referral of private patients. It is worth the GPs' while to shepherd patients towards the private sector if it saves their budgets, and it is worth the consultants' while to encourage them – even if, as the neurologist explained, the diagnostic process might sometimes benefit from the greater periods of waiting that are necessarily endured by NHS patients. Moreover, the occasional practice of offering up private patients to important consultants in return for their preferential handling of NHS patients scarcely suggests an even-handed and equitable management of the waiting list.

A key question, which the interviewees wisely refrained from addressing directly, is whether such effects of rationing eat into the very core of clinical standards, or whether they take their toll at the peripheries of care, in matters of comfort and convenience rather than improvement and recovery. The dividing line is, to some extent, arbitrary. When the nurse manager spoke movingly of hospital nurses no longer having the time to hold the hands of patients in the small hours of the night when they are desperate or anxious, was she voicing a concern about clinical standards or merely about the lack of comfort and succour? As she observed, patients do not die simply because the night comfort is withdrawn, but their experiences of being in hospital may be coloured by it. Or again, when delays in serving meals to patients on the wards are such that the food goes cold and dietary supplements need to be given, is this bad clinical care or bad hotel care?

Several examples were offered, however, of rationing that seemed unquestionably to trespass beyond the realms of comfort and convenience into explicit issues of clinical standards. According to the evidence of the nurse manager, the pressures on ward nurses – resulting from, for example, the large numbers of patients on intravenous drugs – were leading to increasingly more errors in the administration of drugs. Risk assessments on newly admitted patients were not always being carried out as thoroughly as they should have been, leading later on to such preventable problems as pressure sores. It was, the nurse manager thought, an issue of safety: something was happening to patients that was deleterious to their health and that would not have happened if the resources had been available to treat them according to the text-book. The surgeon, too, described the way in which safety issues could be swept aside in the rush of admitting new patients, particularly day patients for whom a bed may not immediately be available. Procedures for ensuring that they have had a pre-medication, that their consent has been obtained, that the site of the operation has been marked, and that their last food and drink intake has been recorded, may not be followed to the letter. He added, however, that such errors, where they occur, are very rarely deleterious to the patients. Things may be done in a slightly rushed and undignified way, without all the required safety features always being in place; but patients get their operations in the end, and they are almost always done safely and well.

Perhaps the major effect of rationing, as revealed by the stories, is reflected in the delay and dilution of care. Services, facilities and treatments may be available in principle but in practice they are provided in ways that make it difficult or impossible for patients to access them as quickly or as fully as they would wish. As the commissioning manager put it, patients will get what they need, eventually, but they may have to wait for it; and the process of waiting constitutes a form of rationing. Thus, the health visitor explained that a laundry was available in her district for families with an incontinent person – but only after two weeks, several phone calls, and a bureaucratic chit. If you put up enough hurdles, she said, the demand for a service will fall off. The GP's fund-holding practice offered in vitro fertilization to its patients – but only for two menstrual cycles. The services of the neurologist were available at a district hospital – but as he was not often there, he could not easily be accessed, and patients with pressing neurological problems were likely to be referred instead to physicians, surgeons or ophthalmologists. The district nurse was able to secure night nursing for her cancer patients from the Marie Curie service – but only for three nights a week. She could mobilize the pressure mattresses that had been purchased from public subscription – but not until other patients had finished using them.

A common form of dilution in nursing care was through the mixing of skills and grades: tasks that should be done (or have traditionally been done) by staff of a particular grade are carried out by less qualified or less experienced people. The district nurse spoke of the use of agency nurses unfamiliar with the area and having only a limited experience of the particular demands of community nursing. Lacking the time to go through the daily list in the detail required, the district nurse could sometimes do little more than to send the agency nurse on her way, only to find later that a dressing may not have been done in quite the right way. The nurse manager often found the daily pressures on the wards to be such that they could be managed only by delegating basic care to unqualified staff. Jobs like hygiene and toileting were done by unqualified nursing assistants, affecting the overall care that patients were receiving.

In these and many other ways the clear sense was conveyed by the stories of a health service under constant pressure, with insufficient resources to meet all the needs of all the patients all the time, yet managing always to provide the best possible care with the highest degree of professionalism. As the geriatrician put it, 'it's a question of continual cohorts of patients coming through, and you have just got to try to do the best you can for each of them in turn . . . There's a constant weight of people coming through, and you know that you have got to move them on and out so that you can make space for the next ones who will be coming through the front door'.

Ethics

The absence of ethical frameworks

How were ethics reflected in the stories? From a formal perspective, they weren't. Few of the interviewees spoke explicitly of an ethically informed awareness that they brought to their work and that informed their decisions. Taken as a whole, the stories reveal an almighty gap between the calm and reflective world of the academics, carefully weighing and delineating the nuances of each word they utter, and the rushed and pragmatic world of the ward and the consulting room, where harassed people, working in pressured environments, are required to make a constant stream of quick decisions on the basis of less than perfect information. Indeed, several of the interviewees spoke specifically of the non-theoretical context of their work. The health visitor remarked that, for her, it wasn't a matter of judging whether one set of criteria was ethically superior to another. 'There aren't any criteria', she said, 'I couldn't really tell you how I make these decisions. You just do, don't you?' The district nurse echoed the point: for her, prioritizing her time was 'something that you do on the hoof, really. You do it as you go along – intuitively.'

Other interviewees said much the same thing. The surgeon described his own response to the pressures he encountered as unplanned and non-purposeful. It was, he said, definitely not rationing in the sense of deciding that he was not going to do such-and-such an operation on patients of such-and-such an age because the outlook for them was so poor or because they had brought it on themselves. Rationing as it affected his work was haphazard, random and *ad hoc*. The geriatrician, similarly, rejected the idea that his decisions reflected a carefully worked-out set of principles. In response to the question of whether he consciously tried to allocate his time and resources in relation to the different needs of his patients, his answer was negative. 'The idea that one patient is more in need than another and should therefore get more of the time of the doctor or the nurse or the therapist does not have any great resonance for me. It doesn't actually work like that.'

Even at the higher level of allocating budgets between different service activities, where more time and reflection might have been expected, no more obvious signs of moral rationality were apparent – if by moral rationality we mean decision-making based upon consciously articulated principles or reflective of particular ethical perspectives. The story told by the public health physician of her authority's attempt to draw up a list of surgical exclusions suggested just as much *ad hocery* at this level as at the clinical coal-face. Although setting out initially to base the exclusions on the kind of criteria made explicit in the use of QALYs, the authority was obliged (for reasons both of technical difficulty and of time constraints) to abandon this principled route in favour of a more pragmatic and workable approach. In the end it was forced, quite simply, to ask itself what would be acceptable within the district – a kind of honest muddling through. To describe the authority's approach even as pragmatic would, the public health physician confessed, be a polite way of describing it.

A not too dissimilar story was reported by the commissioning manager: in the absence of specific central guidelines, he described his authority's approach to its own list of exclusions as 'relatively *ad hoc*'. The price to be paid for the failure firmly to grasp this particular nettle was, however, the investment of a good deal of discretionary authority in the local machinery for deciding marginal cases. In the two authorities represented by the commissioning manager and the public health physician, the machinery was one that had been set up earlier for determining extra-contractual referrals (ECRs); but the very fact that it was working in a discretionary environment exposed it to the influence of strong personalities intent on getting their own way. Commenting on his Trust's recent takeover of the local management of psychiatric ECRs, the psychiatrist observed that 'everybody is in favour of general parsimony and particular expenditure – their own, that is!' Whenever he received a request to authorize an ECR, there was, he explained, always some particular reason put forward by the referring doctor as to why this should be an exception to the rule. From a similar angle, the public health physician was upset by the partiality of her health authority in allowing the expenditure of a large sum of money on a terminally ill patient once the authority had been made aware of personal details from the patient's life. This was, for her, quite simply wrong. 'Nobody stood up and said well, if we spend that huge sum of money on this one patient, lots of little old ladies who live somewhere else in the area won't get their hip replacements or whatever it might be. People like them don't have advocates in high places, and I felt very strongly about that.'

The presence of ethical awareness

Yet despite the predominantly pragmatic and discretionary approach to rationing decisions at the levels of both service planning and clinical care, it would be entirely wrong to assume the existence of an ethical void. Quite the reverse: although few of the interviewees were following *explicitly* articulated ethical frameworks, they seemed well able to judge between morally acceptable and morally unacceptable actions and outcomes, even when they themselves were caught up in them. The GP felt moral unease that his patients, backed by the practice's fund, were securing preferential access to the hospital physiotherapy department at the expense of in-patients with possibly greater needs. It offended his understanding of the purpose of the NHS that triage could be influenced by money rather than need. That he was an accomplice to the deal, albeit a reluctant one, was a measure of the competing – but for him overriding – obligation that he felt to secure the best service for his own patients.

There were other examples, too, of an informed ethical awareness in the absence of explicit ethical frameworks. The health visitor was clear about the injustice that could result from rationing by inaccessibility, in which the astute and the persistent were rewarded at the expense of those who lacked the know-how to seek out what they wanted. Those who are put off, she said, will not be the better-educated middle-class families, they will be the poorer families who are under-educated and inarticulate. She was also aware of an ethically questionable bias in her work in giving subconscious priority to families where she felt able to get the best results – families who were most likely to return to normal functioning with some transient support. That, she explained, was the way that rationing worked: if she had to divide her time between two families, she would instinctively give more of it to the one that was likely to make the more progress. But then, surprised by what she had said, she added: 'Gracious, that's a dreadful thing to do. It may not be wrong, but it's definitely discrimination.'

The surgeon, too, expressed his moral concern at the potential for social bias in the innate responsiveness of the service to the pressure exerted upon it by patients. Those who 'push and shove a bit' will often get the best treatment, but they will not be a cross-section of all those waiting to be seen. He recognized it as wrong (albeit, perhaps, unavoidable) that a class bias will ensue through which cases may not always be seen in the order of their clinical urgency. It was the replacement of need by pressure as the determinant of access to secondary care that he saw as wrong. The neurologist, likewise, felt that triage based upon his assessment of the symptomatology in the referral letter was the fair way of ordering the list of patients waiting to see him, because it reflected what he judged to be the severity of each patient's condition. That errors could occur through the misreading or misinterpretation of the letter was of course unfortunate, but it was a matter of quality rather than rationing. That the logic of triage could be overridden by the preferential access of patients paying privately to see him was different, and the neurologist expressed some unease about it. The GP, too, declared himself to be ambivalent about the morality of private medicine in the context of public rationing. He described it as 'a little underhand' that consultants would see patients more quickly if the referring GP was also a reliable source of private consultations.

A similar ethos of ethical awareness was apparent in the stories of those who worked at the higher level of service planning. Although the public health physician described her authority's compilation of the list of exclusions as a 'very pragmatic and *ad hoc*' exercise that was virtually foisted upon it by the exigencies of its financial position, she was nevertheless aware of its deficiencies. For her, the business of determining service priorities ought, in principle, to proceed on the basis of a clearly articulated ethical foundation, even if the realities of life at the coal-face restricted its application. Her own preferred position was utilitarian. Rooted in her experiences of the harshness of rationing in a Russian winter, her story was replete with an understanding of the finiteness of resources and a sensitivity to the opportunity costs of choice. Decisions should be rational, not whimsical or idiosyncratic. For her it was wrong for decisions to be influenced by the media's championing of tragic cases and it was wrong for her health authority to be swayed in their decision by foreknowledge about the personal and family circumstances of an individual patient.

The nurse manager posed much the same issue in classical terms: are we going to do the greatest good for the greatest number, or are we going to think about the individual? It was, she thought, a particularly acute dilemma for doctors who are trained to do what they judge to be right for individual patients but who find themselves increasingly responsible for managing budgets and attaining corporate targets. She herself offered no judgment, but as a matter of observation she thought that most doctors would place the interests of a single *current* patient above those of a collective of *potential* patients. Several of the interviewees were of the view that publicly expressed opinions and preferences should somehow be engaged in the process of choice at this level – not in deciding whether Mr A or Ms B should have the last remaining place on a life-extending treatment but in deciding how resources should be shared out among a range of competing services. 'In the end it's the public who pay my wages', said the public health physician, 'and what I do with their money must be consistent with what they want.' But she also perceived the ethical down-side of her position: 'what if people prefer cuddly little babies to unattractive people with mental illness or learning difficulties? What do we do then? I really don't have an easy answer to that.'

Principles and practices: a necessary tension

There is widespread rationing in health care both at the managerial level of service planning and at the clinical level of patient care. Services and treatments are not being provided, or not being provided in ideal ways, because of limitations in the availability of resources. Different staff working at different levels in the NHS and accountable in different ways for their decisions are having to cope, round the clock, with the perennial gap between supply and demand in health care. They are doing it in all sorts of ways and for all sorts of reasons. Some of the ways in which rationing works, and some of the effects which it produces, are seen – perhaps quite widely – as morally less defensible than others. Meanwhile the ethicists and the theorists, from the safety of their offices, continue to subject the pantechnicon that is the NHS to repeated MOT tests, inevitably finding it wanting in one or other of its rationing mechanisms.

It is difficult to see with any clarity where we should be going from here, yet certain clues can perhaps be glimpsed. It seems clear that the need for rationing, far from abating, will intensify in the face of the growing capacity of medicine to meet the complex needs of an increasingly sophisticated and demanding public. The Viagra story, which burst upon a fascinated world in 1998, is an obvious exemplar of the point; and many more such stories can be expected. Not only that, the locus of decision-making power is likely to shift increasingly away from the clinical culture of the doctor towards the corporate culture of the manager as the health authorities and primary care groups, backed by the imprimatur of the National Institute for Clinical Excellence, acquire a greater say in what is done and how it is done (Hunter, 1997). At the same time, it seems rather unlikely that public spending on the NHS in the UK will depart dramatically from the steady upward path it has pursued for 50 years. In the 1980s the NHS consumed about 5 per cent of the nation's gross domestic product and in the 1990s about 6 per cent, placing the UK well down the list of developed countries in their overall spending on health (Office of Health Economics, 1997). Dramatic departures from such a trajectory are unlikely to occur, at least in the short term. Continuing efforts to improve the productive efficiency of the NHS, to reduce waste, to target resources on effective treatments and to invest in public health may all ease the difficulties, but they will not close the gap. A radical option in this situation might be to rethink the funding base of health care in Britain, reducing its reliance on public funds and facilitating a greater inflow of private consumer spending through some kind of insurance mechanism; but apart from the encouragement of private capital investment in the NHS, such a move is not even on the agenda of permissible public debate.

It seems clear, also, that no morally 'correct' solutions exist to the problems of rationing in health care systems. This is not to say that possible solutions do not exist (as the earlier chapters in this book have amply shown), merely that no solution has yet emerged which is practicable and which can command unanimous – or even very substantial – professional, political and public support for the values it embodies. If there were such a solution, it would by now be known. Different ways of handling the gap between supply and demand invoke different principles; and principles invoke values; and values are by their very nature pluralist and contested. It could not be otherwise. If we could all agree upon the values that should underlie the disposition of health care resources, much of the contemporary debate about rationing would be greatly simplified; but to suppose that we could ever reach a workable consensus may be a fantasy.

Not only is the search for a morally correct solution to the problem of rationing a chimera, so too must be the belief that a consensual solution, were it ever to be found, would be technically feasible. The very notion of a 'morally correct solution' must imply a standard method of making decisions which can be followed in a more or less uniform way throughout the NHS. Yet if the evidence set out in this book has shown anything, it must be the extreme difficulty, amounting perhaps to the frank impossibility, of ever putting such a project in train. Doctors and other clinicians appear far too absorbed in coping with the welter of daily demands that are made upon them to be able to organize their work within a consistent and consciously articulated ethical framework. Whether or not the tactic of muddling through – even a sensitive and intelligent kind of muddling through – is thought to be desirable, it does seem to accord with the reality of how things are done at the coalface. A strong argument can therefore be made that recognizable links must be forged and maintained between morality and feasibility; it is difficult to see the value of a moral code that is, quite simply, unworkable. The discourses about what is right and what is feasible must keep in step with each other.

For the time being, then, we may simply have to accept that however the rationing processes may work in practice, and whatever the outcomes they produce, they will offend someone's notions of right and wrong. Some people and groups and interests are bound to feel offended or betrayed. That is how the world is. This is not, however, to argue for a kind of moral nihilism. The improbability of finding a consensual moral solution to pressing public problems does not allow us to set aside our moral sensibilities. Quite the reverse. In the case of health care rationing, it is clear that moral questions can and must be asked about the right and the wrong ways of deciding who gets what care. The fact that no agreed or unambiguous answers are likely to emerge does not absolve us from the continuing responsibility of trying to identify and do the least wrong things. And we are not starting with a wholly clean slate. Some of the building blocks are already in place. There does appear to be a certain measure of agreement upon which the debate can build. Nobody, for example, is publicly arguing the righteousness of allowing gender or ethnicity or social status or sexual attractiveness to trump clinical need in a triage mechanism that determines the order in which people are seen and treated. Nobody is publicly defending a system in which NHS patients are used as pawns in the private market for secondary care. Simply to ensure that these relatively simple values are observed and policed would be a positive moral step that few would probably challenge.

Beyond that lie the decisions which may increasingly be forced upon the health authorities and primary care groups about the treatments, procedures and drugs that they will and will not purchase, and beyond that the daily mass of clinical decisions about the ordering, the quantity and the quality of treatments. What has changed here in recent years is the increasingly public gaze beneath which they are taken. Through many different media, including the press, broadcasting and academic publications, the general public is becoming increasingly aware of how the tensions inherent in Weale's (1998) notion of the inconsistent triad are being played off against each other. Such an opening-up of the debate is a good thing. As we noted in the Introduction, to limit the debate about health care rationing only to the *cognoscenti* is to restrict the range of values it can encompass. Health care rationing is liable to affect us all at some point in our lives, and we all have a stake in the debate about how it should – and even more importantly should not – be done. We cannot expect either a consensual or a universally applicable answer to emerge, but we can expect and should demand from government an open and honest account of what the NHS can and cannot afford to provide, and the ways in which the processes of rationing operate at different levels in the service. Whether 'the public' then wish to engage in moral discourse about the ways in which it *should* be done is up to them: as Hunter (1997) shrewdly points out, it is difficult to find any other major areas of government policy where this kind of debate, beloved of democratic theorists, actually occurs. But without an initial openness by government, even the possibility of informed moral discussion is muted.

References

Aaron, H. J. and Schwartz, W. B. (1983) *The Painful Prescription. Rationing Hospital Care*. Washington DC: The Brookings Institution.

Academy of Royal Medical Colleges, British Medical Association, National Association of Health Authorities and Trusts and the National Health Service Executive (1997) *Setting Priorities in the NHS*. London: Academy of Royal Medical Colleges, British Medical Association, National Association of Health Authorities and Trusts and the National Health Service Executive.

Alberti, K. G. G. M. and Lessof, M. (1997) 'Call for council on health priorities' [letter], *The Times*, December 26.

Anon. (1985) 'Rationing of resources', *British Medical Journal*, 290, pp. 374–5.

Arras, J. D. (1997) 'Nice story, but so what? Narrative and justification in ethics', in *Stories and Their Limits. Narrative Approaches to Bioethics* (ed. H. L. Nelson), pp. 65–88. London: Routledge.

Ashmore, M., Mulkay, M. and Pinch, T. (1989) *Health and Efficiency: a Sociology of Health Economics*. Milton Keynes: Open University Press.

Audit Commission (1996) *What the Doctor Ordered: A Study of GP Fundholders in England and Wales*. London: HMSO.

Beauchamp, T. L. and Childress, J. F. (1989) *Principles of Biomedical Ethics*. Oxford: Oxford University Press.

Benzeval, M., Judge, K. and Whitehead, M. (1995) *Tackling Inequalities in Health. An Agenda for Action*. London: King's Fund.

Berger, J. and Mohr, J. (1967) *A Fortunate Man*. London: The Penguin Press.

Berwick, D., Hiatt, H., Janeway, P. and Smith, R. (1997) 'An ethical code for everyone in health care', *British Medical Journal*, 315, pp. 1633–4.

Best, R. (1995) 'The housing dimension', in *Tackling Inequalities in Health. An Agenda for Action* (eds. M. Benzeval, K. Judge and M. Whitehead), pp. 51–68. London: King's Fund.

Bowditch, G. (1997) 'Drugs girl, 15, died after transplant was refused', *The Times*, January 24.

Bowie, C., Richardson, A. and Sykes, W. (1995) 'Consulting the public about health service priorities', *British Medical Journal*, 311, pp. 1155–8.

Bowling, A. (1993) *What People Say about Prioritising Health Services*. London: King's Fund Centre.

Bowling, A. (1996) 'Health care and rationing: the public's debate', *British Medical Journal*, 312, pp. 670–4.

Bradshaw, J. (1972) 'A taxonomy of social need', in *Problems and Progress in Medical Care* (ed. G. McLachlan), pp. 69–82. London: Oxford University Press, for The Nuffield Provincial Hospitals Trust.

Brahams, D. (1985) 'When is discontinuation of dialysis justified?', *The Lancet*, 1, pp. 176–7.

Braine, J. (1957) *Room at the Top*. London: Eyre and Spottiswood.

British Medical Association (1997) *BMA Annual Report of Council 1996–97*. London: British Medical Association.

Buchanan, A. (1980) 'A critical introduction to Rawls' theory of justice', in *John Rawls' Theory of Social Justice* (ed. H. G. Blocker and E. H. Smith). Athens, Ohio: Ohio University Press.

Butler, J. R. (1979) 'Scottish paradox: more doctors, worse health', *British Medical Journal*, 1, 1005–6.

Calabresi, G. and Bobbitt, P. (1978) *Tragic Choices*. New York: W. W. Norton.

Calman, K. (1997) 'Equity, poverty and health for all', *British Medical Journal*, 314, pp. 1187–91.

Carson, D. (1987) 'Baby Barber rocks the legal boat', *The Health Service Journal*, 5079, p. 1403.

Charnley, M. C., Lewis, P. A. and Farrow, S. C. (1989) 'Choosing who shall not be treated in the NHS', *Social Science and Medicine*, vol. 28, 12, pp. 1331–8.

Chinitz, D., Shavel, C., Galai, N. and Israeli, A. (1998) 'Israel's basic basket of health services: the importance of being explicitly implicit', *British Medical Journal*, 317, pp. 1005–7.

Coast, J. (1997) 'Rationing within the health service should be explicit. The case against', in *Rationing. Talk and Action in Health Care* (ed. B. New), pp. 149–56. London: King's Fund and BMJ Publishing Group.

Coast, J., Donovan, J. L. and Frankel, S. J. (1996). *Priority Setting: The Health Care Debate*. Chichester: John Wiley and Sons.

Cochrane, A. L. (1972) *Effectiveness and Efficiency*. London: The Nuffield Provincial Hospitals Trust.

Collee, J. (1995) 'Dr John Collee on the dangers of media appeals to save sick children's lives', *The Observer (Life)*, July 2.

Coote, A. (1997) 'Possibilities for direct public involvement in rationing decisions', in *Rationing. Talk and Action in Health Care* (ed. B. New), pp. 158–64. London: King's Fund and BMJ Publishing Group.

Coote, A. and Lehaghan, J. (1997) *Citizens' Juries: Theory into Practice*. London: Institute of Public Policy Research.

Coulter, A. (1995) 'General practice fundholding: time for a cool appraisal', *British Journal of General Practice*, 45, pp. 119–20.

Crawshaw, R. (1994) 'The Hippocratic oath', *British Medical Journal*, 309, p. 952.

Culyer, A. J. (1976) *Need and the National Health Service*. London: Martin Robertson.

Daniels, N. (1985) *Just Health Care*. Cambridge: Cambridge University Press.

Daniels, N. (1988) *Am I My Parents' Keeper? An Essay on Justice between the Young and the Old*. Oxford: Oxford University Press.

Daniels, N., Light, D. W. and Caplan, R. L. (1996). *Benchmarks of Fairness for Health Care Reform*. Oxford: Oxford University Press.

Danish Council of Ethics. (1996) *Priority-setting in the Health Service – a Report*. Copenhagen: Danish Council of Ethics.

Darwin, C. (1894) *The Descent of Man*. London: John Murray.

Darwin, C. (1985) *The Origin of Species by means of Natural Selection* (ed. J. W. Burrow). London: Penguin Classics.

Day, P. and Klein, R. (1987) 'Accountabilities', in *Five Public Services*. London: Tavistock Publications.

Dean, M. (1991) 'Tobacco deaths versus free speech', *The Lancet*, 338, pp. 1383–4.

Dean, M. (1994) 'Rationing care by age deemed unfair', *The Lancet*, 343, p. 1278.

Dean, M. (1995) 'British health rationing becomes explicit', *The Lancet*, 346, p. 1415.

Delamothe, T. (1994) 'The Hippocratic oath', *British Medical Journal*, 309, p. 953.

Department of Health (1992) *The Health of the Nation. A Strategy for Health in England*. London: HMSO, Cm 1986.

Department of Health (1994) *Being Heard. The Report of a Review Committee on NHS Complaints Procedures*. London: HMSO.

Department of Health (1995) *Government Response to the First Report of the Health Committee, Session 1994–95. Priority Setting*. London: HMSO, Cm 2826.

Department of Health (1997a) *The New NHS. Modern. Dependable*. London: HMSO.

Department of Health (1997b) *On the State of the Public Health 1996*. London: HMSO.

Department of Health (1997c) *Health Action Zones: Invitation to Bid*. London: Department of Health.

Department of Health (1998) *Our Healthier Nation. A Contract for Health*. London: HMSO, Cm 3852.

Department of Health and Social Security (1976a) *Priorities for Health and Personal Social Services in England. A Consultative Document*. London: HMSO.

Department of Health and Social Security (1976b) *Sharing Resources for Health in England*. London: HMSO.

Department of Health and Social Security (1977) *Priorities in the Health and Social Services. The Way Forward*. London: HMSO.

Department of Health and Social Security (1987) *Cash Limits Exposition Booklet 1987/88*. London: HMSO.

Dixon, J. (1992) 'US health care I: The access problem', *British Medical Journal*, 305, pp. 817–19.

Dixon, J. and Welch, H. G. (1991) 'Priority setting: lessons from Oregon', *The Lancet*, 337, pp. 891–4.

Donabedian, A. (1980) *The Definition of Quality and Approaches to its Assessment*. Ann Arbor: Health Administration Press.

Dowling, B. (1997) 'Effect of fundholding on waiting times: database study', *British Medical Journal*, 315, pp. 290–2.

Doyal, L. (1993) 'The role of the public in health care rationing', *Critical Public Health*, 4, pp. 49–52.

Doyal, L. (1995) 'Needs, rights and equity: moral quality in healthcare rationing', *Quality in Health Care*, 4, pp. 273–83.

Doyal, L. (1997a) 'Rationing within the health service should be explicit. The case for', in *Rationing. Talk and Action in Health Care* (ed. B. New), pp. 139–47. London: King's Fund and BMJ Publishing Group.

Doyal, L. (1997b) 'The moral boundaries of public and patient involvement', in *Rationing. Talk and Action in Health Care* (ed. B. New), pp. 171–80. London: King's Fund and BMJ Publishing Group.

Doyal, L. and Gough, L. (1991) *A Theory of Human Need*. Basingstoke: Macmillan.

Draper, P., Best. G. and Dennis, J. (1976) *Health, Money and the National Health Service*. London: Unit for the Study of Health Policy, Guy's Hospital Medical School.

Drever, F. and Whitehead, M. (1997) *Health Inequalities. Decennial supplement*. London: Office for National Statistics.

Dunning, A. J. (1992) *Report of the Government Committee on Choices in Health Care*. Rijswijk: The Netherlands, Ministry of Welfare and Cultural Affairs.

Edwards, B. (1993) *The National Health Service. A Manager's Tale 1946–1992*. London: The Nuffield Provincial Hospitals Trust.

Entwistle, V. A., Watt, I. S., Bradbury, R. and Pehl, L. J. (1996) 'The media and the message. How did the media cover the child B case?' in *Sense and Sensibility in Health Care* (ed. M. Marinker), pp. 87–141. London: BMJ Publishing Group.

Farnham, D. and Horton, S. (eds) (1993) *Managing the New Public Services*. Basingstoke: The Macmillan Press.

Foster, P. (1979) 'The informal rationing of primary medical care', *Journal of Social Policy*, 8, pp. 489–508.

Frank, A. (1995) *The Wounded Storyteller*. Chicago: University of Chicago Press.

Frankel, S. and West, R. (1993) *Rationing and Rationality in the National Health Service*. London: Macmillan.

Fuchs, V. R. (1974) *Who Shall Live? Health, Economics and Social Choice*. New York: Basic Books.

General Medical Council (1995) *Duties of a Doctor: Guidance from the General Medical Council*. London: General Medical Council.

George, V. and Miller, S. M. (1994) *Social Policy towards 2000: Squaring the Welfare Circle*. London: Routledge.

Gilbert, R. (1998) 'Experiences and future visions of the NHS: a younger doctor's perspective', in *Our NHS. A Celebration of 50 Years* (ed. G. Macpherson), pp. 66–70. London: BMJ Books.

Gillon, R. (1985a) 'Justice and medical ethics', *British Medical Journal*, 291, pp. 201–2.

Gillon, R. (1985b) 'Justice and allocation of medical resources', *British Medical Journal*, 291, pp. 266–8.

Gillon, R. (1994) 'Medical ethics: four principles plus attention to scope', *British Medical Journal*, 309 pp. 184–8.

Glaser, W. A. (1970) *Paying the Doctor. Systems of Remuneration and their Effects*, Baltimore: The Johns Hopkins Press.

Griffiths, L. and Hughes, D. (1994) 'Innocent parties and disheartening experiences: natural rhetorics in neuro-rehabilitation admissions conferences', *Qualitative Health Research*, 4, pp. 385–410.

Grimley Evans, J. (1995) 'Equity or equality?', *Journal of the Royal College of Physicians of London*, vol. 29, 3, pp. 186–7.

Grimley Evans, J. (1997) 'Rationing health care by age. The case against', in *Rationing. Talk and Action in Health Care* (ed. B. New), pp. 115–21. London: King's Fund and BMJ Publishing Group.

Gudex, C. and Kind, P. (1988) *The QALY Toolkit*. York: University of York Centre for Health Economics, Discussion Paper 38.

Hadorn, D. C. and Holmes, A. C. (1997) 'The New Zealand priority criteria project', in *Rationing. Talk and Action in Health Care* (ed. B. New), pp. 183–201. London: King's Fund and BMJ Publishing Group.

Ham, C. (1993) 'Priority setting in the NHS: reports from six districts', *British Medical Journal*, 307, pp. 435–8.

Ham, C. and Hill, M. (1984) *The Policy Process in the Modern Capitalist State*. Hemel Hempstead: Harvester Wheatsheaf.

Hampton, J. R. (1983) 'The end of clinical freedom', *British Medical Journal*, 287, pp. 1237–8.

Hansson, L. F., Norheim, O. F. and Ruyter, K. W. (1994) 'Equality, explicitness, severity and rigidity: the Oregon Plan evaluated from a Scandinavian perspective', *Journal of Medicine and Philosophy*, 19, pp. 343–66.

Harman, G. (1977) *The Nature of Morality*. Oxford: Oxford University Press.

Harris, J. (1987) 'QALYfying the value of life', *Journal of Medical Ethics*, 13, pp. 117–23.

Harrison, S. and Hunter, D. J. (1994) *Rationing Health Care*. London: Institute for Public Policy Research.

Harris, J. (1985) *The Value of Life*. London: Routledge and Kegan Paul.

Heginbotham, C. (1997) 'Why rationing is inevitable in the NHS', in *Rationing. Talk and Action in Health Care* (ed. B. New), pp. 43–57. London: King's Fund and BMJ Publishing Group.

Hemingway, H. and Jacobson, B. (1995) 'Queues for cure?', *British Medical Journal*, 310, pp. 818–19.

Hoffenberg, R. (1987) *Clinical Freedom*. London: The Nuffield Provincial Hospitals Trust.

Holm, S. (1998) 'Goodbye to the simple solutions: the second phase of priority setting in health care', *British Medical Journal*, 317, pp. 1000–1002.

Honigsbaum, F., Holmström, S. and Calltorp, J. (1997) *Making Choices for Health Care*. Abingdon: Radcliffe Medical Press.

Horner, J. S. (1996) 'Christian values in medicine', in *Christian Values* (eds E. Stourton and F. Gumley), pp. 94–116. London: Hodder and Stoughton.

Houghton, A. and Hopkins, A. (1996) 'Acute medical admissions: results of a national audit', *Journal of the Royal College of Physicians of London*, 6, pp. 551–9.

House of Commons Health Committee (1995) *Priority Setting in the NHS: Purchasing*. London: HMSO.

Hughes, D. and Griffiths, L. (1996) '"But if you look at the coronary anatomy. . .": risk and rationing in cardiac surgery', *Sociology of Health and Illness*, 18, pp. 172–97.

Hunter, D. J. (1993) *Rationing Dilemmas in Health Care*. Birmingham: National Association of Health Authorities and Trusts.

Hunter, D. J. (1995) 'Rationing health care: the political perspective', *British Medical Bulletin*, 51, pp. 876–84.

Hunter, D. J. (1997) *Desperately Seeking Solutions*. Harlow: Addison Wesley Longman.

Hurwitz, B. and Richardson, R. (1997) 'Swearing to care: the resurgence in medical oaths', *British Medical Journal*, 315, pp. 1671–4.

Jacobson, B. and Yen, L. (1998) 'Health action zones', *British Medical Journal*, 316, p. 164.

Johnston, L., Calvert, J. and Connett, D. (1998) 'Down's babies denied surgery', *The Observer*, February 22.

Kassirer, J. P. (1998) 'Managing care – should we adopt a new ethic?', *New England Journal of Medicine*, 339, pp. 397–8.

Kitzhaber, J. (1993) 'Prioritising health services in an era of limits: the Oregon experience', *British Medical Journal*, 307, pp. 373–7.

Klein, R. (1993) 'Dimensions of rationing: who should do what?', *British Medical Journal*, 307, pp. 309–11.

Klein, R. (1997) 'Defining a package of healthcare services the NHS is responsible for. The case against', *British Medical Journal*, 314, pp. 506–9.

Klein, R. (1998) 'Puzzling out priorities', *British Medical Journal*, 317, p. 959.

Klein, R., Day, P. and Redmayne, S. (1995) 'Rationing in the NHS: the dance of the seven veils – in reverse', *British Medical Bulletin*, 51, pp. 769–80.

Klein, R., Day, P. and Redmayne, S. (1996) *Managing Scarcity. Priority Setting and Rationing in the National Health Service*. Buckingham: Open University Press.

Klein, R. and Maynard, A. (1998) 'On the way to Calvary', *British Medical Journal*, 327, p. 5.

Kneeshaw, J. (1977) 'What does the public think about rationing? A review of the evidence', in *Rationing. Talk and Action in Health Care* (ed. B. New), pp. 58–76. London: King's Fund and BMJ Publishing Group.

Lalonde, M. (1975) *A New Perspective on the Health of Canadians*. Ottawa: Government of Canada.

Lenaghan, J. (1996) *Rationing and Rights in Health Care*. London: Institute for Public Policy Research.

Leu, R. E. and Schaub, T. (1983). 'Does smoking increase medical care expenditure?', *Social Science and Medicine*, 17, pp. 1907–14.

Light, D. W. (1997) 'The real ethics of rationing', *British Medical Journal*, 315, pp. 112–15.

Limentani, A. E. (1997) *A Certain Sympathy*. PhD Thesis, University of Kent at Canterbury.

Limentani, A. E. (1998) 'An ethical code for everybody in health care', *British Medical Journal*, 316, p. 1458.

Lipsky, M. (1980) *Street-level Bureaucracy*. New York: Russell Sage.

Lockwood, M. (1988) 'Quality of life and resource allocation', in *Philosophy and Medical Welfare* (eds J. M. Bell and S. Mendus), pp. 33–55. Cambridge: Cambridge University Press.

Loomes, G. and McKenzie, L. (1989) 'The use of QALYs in health care decision making', *Social Science and Medicine*, 28, pp. 299–308.

Lubitz, J. D. and Riley, G. F. (1993) 'Trends in Medicare payments in the last year of life', *New England Journal of Medicine*, 328, pp. 1092–6.

McKee, M. and Figueras, J. (1996) 'Setting priorities: can Britain learn from Sweden?', *British Medical Journal*, 312, pp. 691–4.

Malek, M. (1994) *Setting Priorities in Health Care*. Chichester: John Wiley and Sons.

Mallick, N. P. (1993) 'End-stage renal failure', in *Rationing of Health Care in Medicine* (ed. M. Tunbridge), pp. 55–64. London: Royal College of Physicians of London.

Marks, L. and Hunter, D. J. (1998) *The Development of Primary Care Groups: Policy into Practice*. London: the NHS Confederation.

Marmot, M. G. and McDowell, M. E. (1986) 'Mortality decline and widening social inequalities', *The Lancet*, ii, pp. 274–6.

Mason, J., Drummond, M. and Torrance, G. (1993) 'Some guidelines on the use of cost effectiveness league tables',. *British Medical Journal*, 306, pp. 570–2.

Maxwell, R. (1995a) *Rationing Health Care*. London: Churchill Livingstone.

Maxwell, R. (1995b) 'Can we do better?', *British Medical Bulletin*, 51, pp. 941–8.

Maynard, A. (1991) 'Developing the health care market', *The Economic Journal*, 101, pp. 1277–86.

Maynard, A. (1996) 'Warning: explicit language', *Health Service Journal*, 5530, p. 20.

Maynard, A. (1997) 'Evidence-based medicine: an incomplete method for informing treatment choices', *The Lancet*, 349, pp. 126–8.

Mays, N. and Bevan G. (1987) *Resource Allocation in the Health Service*. London: Bedford Square Press.

Mechanic, D. (1977) 'The growth of medical technology and bureaucracy: implications for medical care', *Milbank Memorial Fund Quarterly, Health and Society*, 55, pp. 61–78.

Mechanic, D. (1995) 'Dilemmas in rationing health care services: the case for implicit rationing', *British Medical Journal*, 310, pp. 1655–9.

Midgley, M. (1994) 'Darwinism and ethics', in *Medicine and Moral Reasoning* (eds K. W. M. Fulford, G. Gillett and J. M. Soskice). Cambridge: Cambridge University Press.

Mihill, C. (1993) 'Bottomley denies "hotel" fees on way for patients', *The Guardian*, October 26.

Miller, F. H. and Miller, G. A. H. (1986) 'The painful prescription: a Procrustean perspective?', *The New England Journal of Medicine*, 314, pp. 1383–5.

Mooney, G., Gerard, K., Donaldson, C. and Farrar, S. (1992) *Priority Setting in Purchasing. Some Practical Guidelines*. London: National Association of Health Authorities and Trusts.

Morris, J. N. (1975) *Uses of Epidemiology*. Edinburgh: Churchill Livingstone.

Moss, A. H. and Siegler, M. (1991) 'Should alcoholics compete equally for liver transplantation?', *Journal of the American Medical Association*, 265, pp. 1295–8.

Mullen, P. (1995) *Is Health Care Rationing Really Necessary?* Birmingham: Health Services Management Centre.

Murray, S. A., Tapson, J., Turnbull, L., McCallum, J. and Little, A. (1994) 'Listening to local voices: adapting rapid appraisal to assess health and social needs in general practice', *British Medical Journal*, 308, pp. 698–700.

National Health Service Management Executive (1990) *Contracts for Health Services: Operating Contracts*. London, NHS Management Executive.

National Health Service Management Executive (1992) *Local Voices: The Views of Local People in Purchasing for Health*. London: NHS Management Executive.

Nelson, H. L. (1997) *Stories and Their Limits. Narrative Approaches to Bioethics*. London: Routledge.

New, B. (1996) 'The rationing agenda in the NHS', *British Medical Journal*, 312, pp. 1593–1601.

New, B. (1997) 'Defining a package of healthcare services the NHS is responsible for. The case for', *British Medical Journal*, 314, pp. 503–5.

New, B. and Le Grand, J. (1996) *Rationing in the NHS. Principles and Pragmatism*. London: King's Fund Publishing.

Newdick, C. (1995) *Who Should We Treat? Law, Patients and Resources in the NHS*. Oxford: Clarendon Press.

Newdick, C. (1998). 'Primary care groups and the right to prescribe', *British Medical Journal*, 317, pp. 1361–4.

Nord, E. (1992) 'An alternative to QALYs: the saved young life equivalent (SAVE)', *British Medical Journal*, 305, pp. 875–7.

Nozick, R. (1974) *Anarchy, State and Utopia*. Oxford: Basil Blackwell.

O'Dowd T. (1988) 'Five years of heartsink patients in general practice', *British Medical Journal*, 297, pp. 528–30.

Office of Health Economics (1997) *Compendium of Health Statistics, 10th Edition*. London: Office of Health Economics.

Opie, I and Opie. P. (1959) *The Lore and Language of Schoolchildren*. Oxford: Clarendon Press.

Øvretreit, J. A. (1997) 'Managing the gap between demand and publicly affordable health care in an ethical way', *European Journal of Public Health*, 7, pp. 128–35.

Parker, R. A. (1975) 'Social administration and scarcity', in *Social Welfare in Modern Britain* (eds E. Butterworth and R. Holman), pp. 204–12. Glasgow: Fontana Collins.

Pencheon, D. (1998) 'NHS Direct', *British Medical Journal*, 317, pp. 1026–7.

Plamenatz, J. (1966) *The English Utilitarians*. Oxford: Basil Blackwell.

Pollock, A. M. (1992) 'Local voices. The bankruptcy of the democratic process', *British Medical Journal*, 305, pp. 535–6.

Porter, R. (1997) *The Greatest Benefit to Mankind. A Medical History of Humanity from Antiquity to the Present*. London: HarperCollins.

Powell, J. E. (1966) *A New Look at Medicine and Politics*. London: Pitman Medical Publishing.

Powell, M. A. (1997) *Evaluating the National Health Service*. Buckingham: Open University Press.

Price, D. (1996) 'Lessons for health care rationing from the case of child B', *British Medical Journal*, 312, pp. 167–9.

Priestman, T. J., Bullimore, J. A., Goddern, T. P. and Deutsch, G. P. (1989) 'The Royal College of Radiologists Fractionation Study', *Clinical Oncology*, 1, pp. 63–6.

Rawls, J. (1971) *A Theory of Justice*. Cambridge, Mass.: Harvard University Press.

Redmayne, S. (1996) *Small Steps, Big Goals*. Birmingham: National Association of Health Authorities and Trusts.

Rivett, G. (1998) *From Cradle to the Grave. Fifty Years of the NHS*. London: King's Fund.

Roberts, C. (1995) 'Rational rather than rationed', *Health Service Journal*, 5464, p. 17.

Roberts, C. (1996) 'The wasted millions', *Health Service Journal*, 5524, pp. 24–7.

Ross, D. (1966) *The Nicomachean Ethics of Aristotle*. Oxford: Oxford University Press.

Rosser, R. and Kind, P. (1978) 'A scale of values of states of illness: is there a social consensus?', *International Journal of Epidemiology*, 7, pp. 347–58.

Rosser, R. and Watts, V. C. (1972) 'The measurement of hospital output', *International Journal of Epidemiology*, 1, pp. 361–8.

Rous, E., Coppel, A., Haworth, J. and Noyce, S. (1996) 'A purchaser experience of managing new expensive drugs: interferon beta', *British Medical Journal*, 313, pp. 1195–6.

Royal College of Physicians (1995) *Setting Priorities in the NHS: A Framework for Decision Making*. London: Royal College of Physicians of London.

Royal College of Physicians (1998) *Improving Quality in Cancer Care: The Current Role of Paclitaxel in the First-line Chemotherapy of Ovarian Cancer*. London: Royal College of Physicians of London.

Royal Commission on the National Health Service (1979) *Report*. London: HMSO, Cmnd 7615.

Sabin, J. E. (1998) 'Fairness as a problem of love and heart: a clinician's perspective on priority setting', *British Medical Journal*, 317, pp. 1002–4.

Sacket, D. L., Rosenberg, W. M. C., Muir Gray, J. A., Haynes, R. B. and Scott Richardson, W. (1996) 'Evidence based medicine: what it is and what it isn't', *British Medical Journal*, 312, pp. 71–72.

Scrivens, E. (1979) 'Towards a theory of rationing', *Social Policy and Administration*, 13, pp. 53–64.

Shaw, G. B. (1939) *The Doctor's Dilemma: A Tragedy*. London: Constable and Company.

Sheldon, T. (1995) 'Keep taking the Pill . . .', *Health Service Journal*, 5479, pp. 14–15.

Singer, P. (1994) *Ethics*. Oxford: Oxford University Press.

Smith, A. (1987) 'Qualms about QALYs', *The Lancet*, i, pp. 1134–6.

Smith, R. (1991a) 'Where is the wisdom . . .?', *British Medical Journal*, 303, pp. 798–9.

Smith, R. (1991b) 'Rationing: the search for sunlight', *British Medical Journal*, 303, pp. 1561–2.

Smith, R. (1993) *Rationing in Action*. London: BMJ Publishing.

Smith, R. (1996a) 'Being creative about rationing', *British Medical Journal*, 312, pp. 391–2.

Smith, R. (1996b) 'Rationing health care: moving the debate forward', *British Medical Journal*, 312, pp. 1553–4.

Spanjer, M. (1995) 'Changes in Dutch health-care', *The Lancet*, 345, pp. 50–51.

Stacey, M. (1992) *Regulating British Medicine – the General Medical Council*. Chichester: John Wiley.

Stewart, J., Honigsbaum, F., Richards, J. and Lockett, T. (1995) *Priority Setting in Action – Purchasing Dilemmas*. Birmingham: Health Services Management Centre.

Strosberg, M. A., Wiener, J. M., Baker, R. and Fein, I. A. (eds) (1992) *Rationing America's Medical Care: The Oregon Plan and Beyond*. Washington, DC: Brookings Institution.

Taylor-Gooby, P. and Lawson, R. (eds) (1993) *Markets and Managers*. Buckingham: Open University Press.

The Lancet (1998) 'First lessons from the "Bristol case"', *The Lancet*, 351, p. 1669.

The Times (1993) August 18.

The Times (1995) October 12.

The Times (1997) July 12.

The Times Law Report (1995) March 15.

Townsend, P. and Davidson, N. (1982) *Inequalities in Health*. London: Penguin Books.

Tunbridge, M. (ed.) (1993) *Rationing of Health Care in Medicine*. London: Royal College of Physicians of London.

Veatch, R. M. (1992) 'The Oregon experiment: needless and real worries', in *Rationing America's Medical Care: The Oregon Plan and Beyond* (eds M. A. Strosberg, J. M. Wiener, R. Baker and I. A. Fein). Washington, DC: Brookings Institution.

Warnock, M. (1998) *An Intelligent Person's Guide to Ethics*. London: Duckworth.

Watt, I. S. and Entwistle, V. A. (1996) 'What are the implications of the Child B case for the debate on health care policies?', in *Sense and Sensibility in Health Care* (ed. M. Marinker), pp. 142–57. London: BMJ Publishing Group.

Weale, A. (1990) 'The allocation of scarce medical resources: a democrat's dilemma', in *Medicine, Medical Ethics and the Value of Life* (ed. P. Byrne). Chichester: John Wiley.

Weale, A. (1995) 'The ethics of rationing', *British Medical Bulletin*, vol. 51, 4, pp. 831–41.

Weale, A. (1998) 'Rationing health care', *British Medical Journal*, 316, p. 410.

Webster, C. (1988) *The Health Services since the War. Volume 1*. London: HMSO.

Weir, S. and Hall, W. (1994). *Ego Trip. Extra-governmental Organisations in the United Kingdom and Their Accountability*. London: The Charter 88 Trust.

Whitehead, M. (1994) 'Is it fair? Evaluating the equity implications of the NHS reforms', in *Evaluating the NHS Reforms* (eds R. Robinson and J. Le Grand), pp. 208–42. London: King's Fund Institute.

Wilkinson, R. (1996) *Unhealthy Societies*. London: Routledge.

Williams, A. (1997) 'Rationing health care by age. The case for', in *Rationing. Talk and Action in Health Care* (ed. B. New), pp. 108–13. London: King's Fund and BMJ Publishing Group.

Winslow, G. (1982) *Triage and Justice*. Berkeley: University of California Press.

Yates, J. (1995) *Private Eye, Heart and Hip*. Edinburgh: Churchill Livingstone.

Young, J., Robinson, J. and Dickinson, E. (1998) 'Rehabilitation for older people', *British Medical Journal*, 316, pp. 1108–9.

Zimmern, R. (1995) 'Insufficient to simply be efficient', *Health Service Journal*, 5467, p. 19.

Index